Praise for
Chains, Whips, and Cuffs

"Rev Jen's *BDSM 101* provides the helpful tips, witty insights, and important safety information that anyone new to—or even just interested in—BDSM needs to know. It's a great starter manual for anyone interested in moving from reading *Fifty Shades of Grey* to actually living it out." —Lux Alptraum, editor of Fleshbot.com

"Everything you need to know to know about BDSM and only the way Rev. Jen could tell it. Quirky, witty, intelligent, entertaining, and hilariously dirty. I had to flog myself several times while reading it. If you don't know what that is, you definitely need to read this book!" —Ruby LaRocca, actress and scream queen extraordinaire

"If you want to know what to do with rope, clothespins, handcuffs, dirty words and much more, look no further than Reverend Jen's helpful and humorous guide to the ins and outs of BDSM. Her tell-it-like-it-is advice is perfect for the curious kinky newcomer." —Rachel Kramer Bussel, editor, *Best Bondage Erotica 2013*

CHAINS,
WHIPS,
AND CUFFS

CHAINS, WHIPS, AND CUFFS

A Beginner's Guide to
the Ecstasy and Pain of BDSM

by

Rev. Jen

Illustrations by Brian Peterson

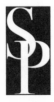

SKYHORSE PUBLISHING, INC.

Skyhorse Publishing books may be purchased in bulk at special discounts for sales promotion, corporate gifts, fund-raising, or educational purposes. Special editions can also be created to specifications. For details, contact the Special Sales Department, Skyhorse Publishing, 307 West 36th Street, 11th Floor, New York, NY 10018 or info@skyhorsepublishing.com.

Skyhorse® and Skyhorse Publishing® are registered trademarks of Skyhorse Publishing, Inc.®, a Delaware corporation.

Visit our website at www.skyhorsepublishing.com.

10 9 8 7 6 5 4 3 2 1

Library of Congress Cataloging-in-Publication Data

Reverend Jen, 1972-
BDSM 101 / Rev. Jen.
192 pages cm

ISBN: 9781510717527
Ebook ISBN: 9781510717534

1. Sexual dominance and submission. 2. Sadomasochism. 3. Bondage (Sexual behavior) I. Title. II. Title: BDSM one hundred one. III. Title: BDSM one hundred and one.
HQ79.R48 2013
306.77'5--dc23

                             2012046067

Cover design by Jane Sheppard

Printed in the United States of America

To Velocity, a glorious hellion

Table of Contents

What is BDSM?
(And how I unintentionally become a sexpert . . .)

1

Safety First!
(It's only funny till someone gets hurt!)

9

Have Fun!

15

What If Your Partner Just Ain't into It?
(And what if you don't have a partner?)

17

A (Very Brief) Glossary of Terms

23

Becoming an Endor-Fan!

29

Types of BDSM Relationships

31

On With the Show!
(The "nuts" and bolts and fun stuff . . .)

37

Talk Dirty to Me!
(*It's not just a bitchin' Poison song...*)

39

Verbal Humiliation

43

Physical Humiliation

49

Spanking

53

Timing

63

Flagellation

65

Fetishes

75

Role-Play

79

Temperature Play

89

Sensation Play

105

Human Bondage!

117

Collars

131

Fisting the Night Away!

139

Into Golden Showers? *Urine Luck!*

143

Behind Enema Lines!

145

Glory HOLEllujah! (*Home Décor for Pervs*)

147

Going Pro

151

Edge Play

153

Therapy and Transcendence

161

The End

167

Acknowledgments

169

What is BDSM?

(And how I unintentionally become a sexpert . . .)

Remember when you were trying to memorize the colors of the rainbow and you learned the acronym ROYGBIV (red, orange, yellow, green, blue, indigo, violet)? BDSM is like the ROYGBIV of kinky sex. The term is a condensed acronym representing practices ranging from bondage and discipline (B&D or B/D), dominance and submission (D&S or D/s), and sadomasochism or sadism and masochism (S&M or S/M). The kinks falling under this umbrella term are many—bondage, whipping, role-play, spanking, strap-on play, cock and ball torture, foot fetishism, hot wax play, blindfolds, and more—a cavalcade of sexual practices as colorful as the rainbow!

Because you have picked up *BDSM 101*, I am guessing you aren't writing a dissertation on the topic nor are you reading this alongside your hog-tied, latex-clad personal slave. This book is intended for beginners, for those who are curious and want to discover what BDSM has to offer. Maybe you and your partner have been banging away in the missionary position for twenty years and just want to spice things up a bit. Maybe you are single and looking to get involved in BDSM. This book will provide you with a solid foundation for doing just that. This is *not* a book for people who are already submerged in the lifestyle, but for those who are curious.

If you think of BDSM as a foreign country that you desperately want to visit, but where you don't speak the language, this book will teach you a few words to get by. Consider this a crash course in the basics and me your nutty professor. Keep in mind I am not a licensed sexologist. Though my qualifications are manifold, they are based largely on my sense of adventure, my libidinous nature, and years of debauched "fieldwork."

My own introduction to BDSM came through literature. As a teen, I was interested in any book deemed obscene; so naturally, I picked up a copy of *Story of O*, a tale of female submission. In it, a beautiful Parisian fashion photographer, O, is brought to a château by her lover René, where she is trained to serve a group of men. She is blindfolded, chained, whipped, branded, pierced, made to wear a mask, and taught to be constantly available for intercourse. It was a novel I read several times, always with one hand. Despite being a feminist, O's objectification turned me on, and a few years later, when I found a boyfriend and we experimented with blindfolds and rope bondage, I discovered why. Surrendering made me feel appreciated and beautiful, if only on the most superficial level. It was the ultimate narcissistic high. And like reading a book many considered filthy, the idea that I was doing something "bad" got me hot.

Still, my sex life remained fairly vanilla until shortly after graduating from art school when I found myself without rent money or marketable skills. Rolling pennies, writing, painting, and doing performance art in rundown art-holes was just not cutting it in terms of a financial plan. I needed a job fast or I would lose my rent-stabilized Manhattan apartment. That's when my friend, Velocity Chyaldd, made a suggestion. Velocity was the front woman for a metal band who also did performance art wherein she simulated knifing her vagina onstage. She suggested I could make some money at the dungeon where she worked. A *dungeon* (sometimes called an S&M/fetish parlor) is a place where men and women (mostly men) pay hundreds of dollars so that dominatrices will dominate them. Sometimes the men and women (again, mostly men) pay hundreds of dollars so they can dominate submissives. Velocity thought I'd make a great submissive. I was twenty-three, had a gamine's body, loose morals, a writer's curiosity, and "an ass made for spanking"—according to her. Plus, I was intrigued.

Though I had no experience in the sex industry and very little experience with BDSM, I got the job, which I accepted without hesitation. Though the sex industry scared me, the thought of eviction scared me more. As a result, I spent the next few years working as a professional submissive, first at the dungeon and then for a woman with a master's degree in human sexuality who founded a company for counseling, erotic role-play, and video production for health-related services.

Finally, when I tired of both the dungeon and the "counseling center" (which was really just a dungeon that offered therapy) taking 50 percent of my profits, I began to do private sessions with another submissive named "Annie" at her Chelsea Hotel pad. We did all our sessions together and only with regulars. Plus, we kept 100 percent of the profits, which meant I worked about five total hours a week while devoting the rest of my time to making art and going nuts—partying, drinking, and screwing an assortment of crazies. (I was in my early twenties, a time when it's almost a crime against nature not to.)

But when all was said and done, I got a lot more "material" than I bargained for. Like O, I was blindfolded, whipped, humiliated, caned, and chained, but the difference was that O had submitted for love and I was doing it for money. It was a *big* difference. I occasionally reached unbelievable heights of sexual ecstasy, but I also spent a lot of time dealing with douche bags. Money changes everything, though not always for the best.

Eventually I quit and found "normal" work in retail. In hindsight, I realize that there were other options I could have explored as a broke twenty-three-year-old, but I didn't. Why I didn't, I'll never know. Maybe it was truly writer's curiosity that led me down this path. What I *do* know is that I chose to traverse the road less traveled and that it was a great learning experience. I got a firsthand look at the fetishes, obsessions, and desires of others and a thorough education in BDSM.

But the adventure didn't end there. Almost a decade after I quit the "industry," *Nerve* offered me an even stranger job writing a column called "I Did It for Science." *Nerve* is an online magazine dedicated to sex, relationships, and culture. Each month, they asked me to perform a new "sexperiment" and then write about it. For the next two years, I exhausted myself performing every deviant act known to man and in the process became an accidental sexpert.

I worked as a live nude girl at Wiggles (a nude strip club), made a sex video, threw a key party like the one in *The Ice Storm*, attended a "balloon fetish party" (wherein I jumped inside a giant balloon), became a nude housecleaner, attended fellatio school, held a Sex Toy Olympics, and more. At one point I attended an S&M academy called Princess Reform School where my graduation entailed being stripped naked at an orgy, chained to a wooden X, blindfolded, caressed by strangers, encased in plumage, and (via the use of a high-speed vibrator) brought to screaming orgasm in front of everyone. It was a BDSM scenario that became a permanent part of my mental spank bank. Yet, despite the fun I had, the column eventually ran its course, though my collected columns led to my first book, *Live Nude Elf*.

When I lost my job at *Nerve*, I didn't even bother looking in the normal help wanted section of the paper. Instead, I but turned immediately to the "adult help wanted" ads. Clearly, I was too insane to get a normal job but too sane to get disability. My search led me to yet another unusual gig—working as a sex surrogate for a renowned sex therapist.

Many people are confused by what sex surrogates actually do. Because the words *sex* and *surrogate* are involved, many people assume surrogates are prostitutes, which they are not. Most surrogates teach through talking, listening, and demonstrating sexual touch. Patients saw the therapist for forty-five minutes of talk therapy before seeing me for forty-five minutes of "physical" therapy. The list of problems I assisted in treating ran the gamut from premature ejaculation to erectile dysfunction and everything in between—inexperience, shyness, vaginal aversion, and inhibited orgasm.

The therapist I worked for advocated the use of sensate focus exercises to overcome these issues. *Sensate focus* is a term that was first introduced by William H. Masters and Virginia E. Johnson and was aimed at increasing personal and interpersonal awareness of self and the other's needs. As a Wikipedia search will reveal, each participant is encouraged to focus on his or her own varied sense experience, rather than to see orgasm as the sole goal of sex. In other words, instead of focusing on whether you're going to blow your load too soon, or blow your load at all, or make your partner blow *their* load, you should just focus on how good sex *feels*. This is a task that's easier said than done given most of the population's anxiety, low self-esteem, reliance on porn, and distractibility. We're all so caught up in what's going on in our heads that we've practically forgotten we have bodies. Exercises I did with patients ranged from simple "hand touching" to actual penis-stroking to teaching men "sexual touch" by first giving them an "anatomy lesson" wherein I displayed my beaver and pointed out the various anatomical "parts." None of this bothered me. In fact, the idea of helping hordes of men find the clit thrilled me. I nicknamed the therapy center Dick School and considered myself one of its greatest teachers.

Work at Dick School was fulfilling and I stayed until my boss retired, less than two years after I started. When first hired, she had promised me I would change lives—and I did. Maybe I wasn't going to win a Nobel Prize for my work there, but I helped many patients overcome seemingly insurmountable problems in order to finally experience pleasure. And at the end of the day, the more people who experience pleasure on this planet, the better.

Keep this in mind as you read along. Happy, fucking people with awesome sex lives are part of the solution, not part of the problem. (Except for the overpopulation problem.) Aside from that, happily fucking people are far less likely to blow shit up and randomly kill people than those who aren't fucking happily. Just by reading this manual—by attempting to spice up your love life and, in the process, make your partner (or partners) excited and joyful—you are making the world a better place. Enjoy the lessons learned herein and pat yourself on the back (or anywhere else you like, should you find them titillating) for making the effort.

And finally, a special shout-out to the laydees. As mentioned previously, I am a feminist. For me, *feminist* simply means you believe women should have the same rights as men, which sadly, they don't. Atrocities are committed against girls and women in every corner of the globe every day (and against the greatest Mother of all—Earth . . . Guess I just came out as a pagan goddess-worshipping hippie as well as a feminist). I mention this because of the book *Fifty Shades of Grey*, which it seems roughly a gazillion people have read and which has spawned newfound interest in BDSM. It's doubtful my mother and I would have ever had a conversation containing the term "butt plug" were it not for the book's publication.

However, since it came out many people have called *Fifty Shades* a backlash against feminism, arguing that the story, one of a female submissive falling for a dominant male, is degrading to women. Sure, it's not highbrow literature, and yes, the female protagonist is naïve while the male character is strong and successful, but these are *fantasy* archetypes and *Fifty Shades* is the S&M equivalent of a Harlequin Romance bodice-ripping novel.

Though part of the fun of BDSM is that you get to act out fantasy archetypes, hopefully anyone who reads *this* book will realize that whether you are submissive or dominant, male or female, gay or straight, the reality of BDSM is that it is a shared experience where both partners are equals. It can be intensely erotic, loving, transcendental, or just plain ol' dirty fun. Regarding BDSM, I'd have to say, "Don't knock it till you've tried it."

I was a female submissive for years, working within the sex industry, and at no point did I feel degraded. It was painful at times and always frustrating because I was still a struggling writer who (much as I love S&M) would have rather been writing than swinging from a suspension bar half-naked. But the lessons I learned and the human connections I made were invaluable.

So please, if you are a female with submissive urges, do not feel like a freak. Do not feel like you are weak or that you are betraying your own sex. (And if you are a dominant male, it does not mean that you hate women; it simply means you have a kink.) So people, let your freak flags fly. If you practice BDSM in a safe, sane, consensual manner, you are simply courageous sexual explorers.

Safety First!
(*It's only funny till someone gets hurt!*)

If one were to liken this book to a fitness video, this would be the part at the beginning where the celebrity trainer tells viewers that before this or any other workout, they should consult a doctor. Given how many of us don't actually have health insurance, a doctor's visit could prove impossible. But try to make sure you're in halfway decent shape before engaging in any of the earth-shattering acts described on the following pages. I don't want anyone reading this book and suffering a heart attack from overexertion. If you are with a new partner, ask if they have any preexisting conditions such as epilepsy, a bad back, or a weak heart. The last thing you want is someone pulling a Nelson Rockefeller on your ass.

> ### Necessary Disclaimer:
>
> Nobody associated with the writing, publication, sale, or distribution of this book is in any way liable for injuries that may result from your engaging in the acts described herein. So be careful for Christ's sake!

Regular sex is risky and BDSM is ten times more so. And if you go to a professional house of domination, *please* let the staff know if you have a preexisting condition. My first week on the job as a sub, one of Velocity's clients had a grand mal seizure (and hadn't told the staff about his condition). Luckily, she knew exactly what to do, remained calm, and called emergency technicians who must've found our dungeon (with its penis-shaped wall hooks, suspension devices, and giant wheels you could strap slaves on) rather odd. Even so, if somebody becomes seriously ill or is in trouble during BDSM play or even regular ol' fucking, don't be too ashamed to call an EMT even if you are buck naked and horrified by whatever scenario is transpiring. *Life* is more important than *pride*—or even that house in Vegas your play partner's wife will likely get after the expensive divorce settlement.

Also, please don't use this guidebook as your only source of information. Do plenty of research on the subject, but also realize that some porn you might come across while "researching" will feature nonconsensual acts such as rape and torture. This is not BDSM! *Real* BDSM is loving, fun, consensual, and, for some, spiritually rewarding.

I've started with safety because practitioners of BDSM follow the mantra "safe, sane, and consensual." This philosophy is important for many reasons. First, you don't want to do anything unsafe (like leaving a partner alone while he or she is tied up) because there's nothing sexy about a 3 AM emergency room visit. And you certainly want to be in a sane frame of mind while engaging in BDSM activities (i.e., not on drugs, wasted, manic, or angry) so you don't say or do something that could damage your relationship or, worse, could endanger your partner's life. And *never* do anything with someone incapable of consent (i.e., wasted and disorderly, on drugs, too mentally ill to give consent, or too young). That is just wrong, immoral, and, in many cases, illegal.

Communication is key when getting kinky, so discuss what's going to happen before the clothes even come off. (It's also a good idea to spend some time afterward discussing what went down, especially if it's with a relatively new partner.) Negotiate boundaries and be sure the sub consents to whatever is going to occur. Like visits to the ER, there's also nothing sexy about a lover sitting on the edge of the bed crying because he or she feels violated. It's important for the Dom to also set boundaries lest he is with a pushy sub who wants him to go too far. As a Dom, *never,* even with the sub's desire and consent, do anything that would recklessly endanger him or her.

If you've read *Fifty Shades of Grey,* you'll remember that even the dominant and dashing Mr. Grey wrote down his "hard limits"—things he absolutely would not do. These included no fire play, no acts involving urination and defecation, and no acts involving needles, piercing, or blood—among others. Think about what your hard limits are, write them down, and share with your partner.

"Soft limits," on the other hand, are limits set by either the Dom or sub that can change if necessary. Sometimes, over the course of a relationship, limits change (e.g. a sub's tolerance for pain), but in the beginning be *very specific*. And always be aware of the difference between BDSM and abuse. *Abuse* is defined as physical, sexual, or emotional acts inflicted on a person without his or her informed and freely given consent. If you have been abused, or if you are considering abusing another in the guise of BDSM, please seek professional help.

Limits and consent are meant to keep a sub safe and to let the Dom know where to draw the line. They also communicate what each partner finds enjoyable and enjoyment is, after all, the goal here.

While working at the dungeon, we kept files on the clients in which they were asked to rate fetishes and preferences on a scale of 1 to 5, 5 being most preferred. Even so, we had to meet with each client beforehand to discuss limits and boundaries. One of the good things about working in a swanky dungeon (that I won't name for reasons of legality) is that they took various safety precautions to save their own asses (and mine).

The dungeon housed different rooms where we did sessions. Thematically and stylistically, they ranged from a French rococo suite to a "medical" room that looked like something out of *Barbarella,* to a plain ol' gloomy medieval dungeon. Like the walls of a haunted mansion on *Scooby Doo,* the walls of each room rotated into the next. It was a secret that only employees were privy to, just in case you had to escape a lunatic. We also had intercoms, which we could use to communicate with the front desk if necessary.

Still, there were moments when I questioned my safety. I once asked a new client what he liked and he responded, "Have you ever been beaten?" I simply walked out. It didn't help that when I walked into the waiting room, he had already removed his clothes and was sitting there in ripped, dirty tighty whities. Plus he had a long, white beard more reminiscent of a maniacal hillbilly than Gandalf. Never do anything that makes you uneasy.

If you happen to be meeting with a new play partner (not recommended, but it happens), make sure you meet with him or her beforehand for some straight time (e.g., a cup of coffee and a chat) before getting down to business and *always* let a trusted friend know what you're up to and where. Tell that friend you will send him or her a text stating that you are safe at a specific hour. If he or she doesn't hear from you, it's cause for concern.

When it comes to safe play, *always* choose a safe word. This is a code word the sub can utter if he or she is in or approaching emotional or physical distress and would like to halt the activity. It's best to choose a simple, memorable word. My first day on the job as a sub, my client said, "We need a safe word. Pick a color."

"Violet," I said, and then thought, *what a stupid safe word.* Who wants to utter three syllables when they're in pain? Plus it sounded too much like "violence." But I could hardly change it, since he certainly wasn't paying me to recite the contents of a box of Crayola.

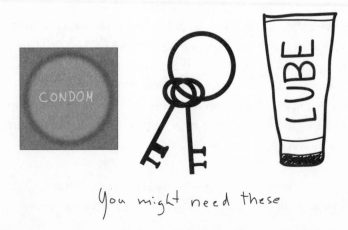

You might need these

My best friend, the performance artist and writer known as Faceboy a.k.a. Francis Hall (who for this book asked to be referred to as "Mr. Hall" because it sounds more dominant), recently told me that he and his girlfriend have three safe words—*red, yellow,* and *green.* Red means "stop completely." Yellow means "slow down," and green means "pleeeease keep going!" Mr. Hall also shared another inventive tip—if your sub is gagged, place a set of keys in his/her hand. Dropping the keys is his/her gagged safe word.

If you are a Dom, remember that sometimes a sub will enter a deep "subspace" (a transcendental state wherein he or she feels as though they are floating and impervious to pain). So it's a good idea to check in with the sub by occasionally asking, "Are you okay?"

Throughout this book, I'll share other safety tips related to each topic. (When we get to flagellation, for example, we'll cover where it's okay to whip someone.) However, no chapter on safety would be complete without mentioning one of mankind's greatest inventions— condoms.*

If you aren't in a trusting, committed relationship where both partners have been tested and "doing it" is going to be part of your play, have plenty of one-piece overcoats handy. Make sure they're not expired and that they're kept in a convenient, memorable location since there's nothing worse than traipsing bare-assed across a room on a condom quest while in the heat of the moment. Next to the condoms, perhaps keep a big bottle o' lube, especially if you are doing any sort of anal play. Remember (as with the condoms) where you've put it. I'm actually considering creating a lube armband after misplacing my Liquid Silk one too many times.

---

*If you live in New York City, we actually have free, official NYC condoms. They're not "ribbed for her pleasure," mint-flavored, studded, or anything fancy, but they work just fine. You can get bags of five hundred from the Gay Men's Health Crisis or simply grab a handful at most bars and clubs. It will save you that uncomfortable trip to the bodega at 2 AM—not to mention your hard-earned cash. In this recession, free condoms are to sex what government cheese is to dairy goodness. Certain clinics like Planned Parenthood also provide free condoms, so go get 'em!

In summation, remember the following lest somebody gets hurt!

1. Negotiate and discuss the scenario beforehand.
2. Set limits.
3. Make sure you and your partner are in a sane frame of mind.
4. Choose a safe word (or three!).
5. Research whatever practices you are about to engage in to ensure you perform them safely.
6. If you are meeting with someone new, let a friend know!
7. Use a raincoat!
8. Don't lose the lube.

Your Turn!

Take a page from *Fifty Shades of Grey*: Define your limits! Use the table below to set your hard and soft limits. Think about what you know you like, what you know you don't, and what you've always wanted to try while you make your lists.

Partner 1		Partner 2	
Hard Limits	Soft Limits	Hard Limits	Soft Limits

Have Fun!

It might seem ridiculous that, in a book about kinky sex, I have written a section titled "Have Fun!"

You are likely wondering, "If people are screwing and spanking and teasing and other good dirty stuff, aren't they already having fun?" Sadly, the answer is "not always."

While working as a surrogate, one of the biggest problems I saw was people who took sex too seriously. Take doing your taxes and paying your bills seriously, but when it comes to sex, loosen up and have fun—especially when you are trying something new like BDSM. There are bound to be awkward moments, so don't be afraid to act silly.

For example . . .

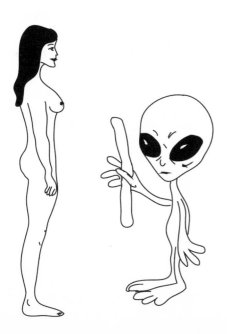

In one exercise I did with patients called The Martian Game, we would strip down to our underwear, keep our eyes closed, and take turns pretending to be either space aliens or explorers of another planet. The aliens would present to the space explorers three body parts, one at a time, and the explorers would have to describe each one, playfully guessing what each part might be used for.

After round one, we'd take off our underwear and do another totally naked round of Martian Game. At this point, if the alien wanted to present to you its penis, it could, and you (the explorer) might guess that it's a prehensile tail or nose or some other kooky alien part. I suppose you could even guess it's a penis.

The point of Martian Game was to teach patients to not get so worked up about things that happen in the bedroom while also encouraging them to continue to focus on sensation. It was not unlike BDSM role-play and it inevitably led to laughter.

I once dated a man with a "female wrestler" fetish. He'd developed it watching *G.L.O.W.* (Gorgeous Ladies of Wrestling) as an adolescent and he wanted me to wear wrestling leotards when we fooled around. I acquiesced and at first felt like a complete moron in my spandex getup, but once I saw how hot it made him, *I* got turned on. And when we started rolling around together, "wrestling," we had a blast, both of us laughing while growing increasingly aroused. It wasn't long before the spandex came off.

Bottom line: Don't worry about "making love like a porn star." Porn stars get paid the big bucks because they are really good at what they do. (And having once been a P.A. on a porn set, I can attest to the fact that they earn every penny.) So let go and have a good time. When two people fuck, they bond. When they can laugh and smile while doing it, even if one of them is having their ass spanked, the bond is even stronger.

What If Your Partner Just Ain't into It?

(And what if you don't have a partner?)

Broaching the Subject with Your Partner

Say you've been fantasizing about BDSM for years and you finally get up the courage to share your fantasies with your partner only to find out he/she just isn't into it. What do you do? The answer is obvious—cheat! (Just kidding.) Honesty is (almost) always the best policy, so tell your partner what you think and feel. This takes courage, but BDSM has recently become more mainstream and (motivational poster time) anything worth doing usually takes courage. I have a magnet on my fridge that says, "Ask for what you want. You just might get it." This is practically a no-fail policy unless you are into something exhausting like being an adult baby or being shat on.

An even *better* policy than honesty is flattery, so be sure to tell your lover how much you'd love to see her gorgeous body tied up or how much you'd love her gorgeous body to tie *you* up. Use the word "beautiful" as often as possible and there shouldn't be a problem. However, don't nag and don't bring up your kink every waking second. It will drive your partner crazy (not in a good way).

You can also broach the subject by watching dirty movies together and making subtle suggestions. Maybe say, "Adrian Lyne is an incredibly underrated director. Let's watch everything he's ever directed including *Nine and ½ Weeks.*" Then, as you watch Mickey Rourke rub ice up and down Kim Bassinger's naked body, you mention, "Hey, this retro '80s behavior is kinda hot. Can you please get some ice out of the freezer?" I cannot imagine this not working.

Maybe you did read *Fifty Shades of Grey* (last time I bring it up, I swear) and it made you moist or heavy. Work up the nerve to say to your partner, "I'd like to be tied up like the chick in *Fifty Shades of Grey*. Let's go to the hardware store and buy some rope." Make it a fun, conspiratorial "field trip" as you both share in the secret knowledge that you are at Home Depot for reasons other than home improvement.

There are also a number of ways you can nonverbally communicate what you'd like to gauge your partner's interest in BDSM, especially during intercourse. If you are dominant, try lightly pinning your partner's hands down as you make love to him or her or try very lightly pulling his or her hair. (*Lightly* is the key word. I still have a pinched nerve from when an inconsiderate lover ambushed me with a surprise hair-pull attack. Made for a somewhat uncomfortable trip to the doctor.) One great method for pulling hair that won't send your partner to a chiropractor is to gently slide your hand up the back of his or her neck, spread your fingers slowly and squeeze the hair close to the scalp. Never yank someone's hair.

If you are submissive, you can gauge your partner's interest in domination by putting your hands above your head while "doing it" to see if he or she pins you down. Other nonverbal hints could be as simple as placing a coil of rope on the nightstand next to the bed or hanging a riding crop from your door.

Ultimately, if your partner is truly your soul mate, you should support whatever decision he or she makes. If your partner isn't into it, you can always fantasize and jack yourself silly on your own time. If your partner happens to be a horrible person, then it might be time to move on and find someone who shares your kink.

Finding Someone New to Play With

In terms of where to meet people with similar kinks, it seems FetLife is the BDSM dating website of choice (the "Facebook of kink") though I've heard (from many hot, horny, kinky people) that they've been unable to find love there.

If you live in a city, maybe just do it the old-fashioned way: go to bars and actually talk to people. This is becoming a rare, lost art, but there are plenty of fetish parties out there just waiting for you. In more populated areas, you can find local clubs devoted to S&M. These are fun—not always sexy but fun. So think of a trip to one as an adventure and keep your expectations low.

For example . . .

Mr. Hall recently told me of a time when he took a lady friend to the Hellfire Club, a (now closed) once popular heterosexual-friendly BDSM club that flourished in New York City's meatpacking district.

"We just weren't ready to see an old man with a tampon up his ass," Mr. Hall explained. "Not to be too full of ourselves but we were the youngest and possibly the hottest couple there, so people started following us around with their dicks out. We weren't turned on, but we didn't want to leave without having some fun. . . .

"So we went into one of the rooms and I turned her towards the wall. Then I just started clapping my hands together so it seemed as if I were spanking her. A large crowd . . . most of the club surrounded us and then I turned around and clapped to them, revealing that there was no spanking at all. We were greeted with a mix of disappointment and dumbfounded silence. Many people put their dicks away."

He added, as an addendum to the story, that he felt shitty about his trickery. "They were mostly nice people," he said. "I went back there many times afterward and had a great, bonerific time."

If you happen to live in a town with a population of forty where everyone is a prude, either get the hell out of dodge or do go online and start doing research.

You might meet someone on the web who shares your fetishes and desires, but with whom you share nothing else. Make sure you have more in common than a butt plug collection before meeting up for a liaison. Nothing will kill desire faster than bad conversation.

Having never dated online (or even "hooked up" with anyone online), I asked my friends for online dating/hook up stories and advice. One friend simply responded, "Do you want the '600 lb guy at the Chinese buffet' story or the 'I'd really like to be in your panties' story? This is why I decided to get married."

But be careful!

If you go online, make sure if you are talking to "Jane," a hot twenty-something who likes bondage, you aren't actually talking to "Ron," a retired plumber who is just fucking with you.

Although this is a book about BDSM and not finding a life partner, wouldn't it be nice to find a partner who you can treat and honor you like a god or goddess outside of the bedroom and like a wild, kinky slut *in* the bedroom? When writing a personal ad, it's best to be totally honest about what you really look like, whether you have any sexually transmitted diseases, addiction issues, or are married with children. In fact, you might even want to send crappy photos of yourself so that when your prospective partner sees how unbelievably beautiful you are in real life, he or she will be blown away.

The descriptions of my friend's failed dates say a lot, but do not despair. After I finish writing this chapter, I'm going to crash the wedding reception of a couple who met on eHarmony. Success stories happen every day, but that doesn't mean you shouldn't be careful in the meantime.

What You Should Have Learned

If you already have a partner, be subtle and honest in your approach. Many people are shy, especially when it comes to sex. Even couples who've been married for twenty years sometimes have trouble communicating what they want, but if you don't ask for what you want, you'll never get it.

If you don't have a partner, take the same approach—one of directness—but be cautious because the world, and especially the Internet, is full of maniacs or worse—boring people!

One last, extremely important bit of advice: If you are married and in a high-profile position of power, don't email or text nekkid or even shirtless pictures of yourself to prospective partners lest you end up jobless, on *TMZ*, and paying alimony out the ass.

A (Very Brief) Glossary of Terms

Before we get started with the par-tay—the chips, dips, chains, and whips—it's important to know the most basic terms.

Again this is a *very brief* glossary. If you go online and Google BDSM, you'll find something akin to what would happen if Merriam-Webster and Urban Dictionary got drunk and made a Bride of Frankenstein. Later we'll get to the tricks and tools of the trade, but here we'll just focus on the participants.

At the dungeon, I noticed two distinct categories. Plenty of my coworkers were *lifestyle Doms.* They practiced their trade at home with their lovers and went to fetish events and fully embraced the fetish lifestyle. Some of the Doms were actually *lifestyle subs* who switched roles once they got home. And then there were girls who were just trying to make a buck, put themselves through college, or simply keep roofs over their heads. Though I'd already experimented with some wild sex acts, I'd originally thought myself the latter. Only later did I realize I'm actually something of a perv, mainly a sub. No one is leading me around by a collar night and day, but I do enjoy light play and have experienced heavy play.

Keep in mind that if you are into BDSM, you are not alone and you are not a freak. I won't throw percentages out there (since estimates vary widely), but a lot of people dig it. I'm guessing there are more people into BDSM than the entire population of South Dakota . . . or maybe even North Dakota and probably even some small countries. Point is—I am not Masters or Johnson, but I *do* know BDSM has been around for a long time and is extremely popular. It is mentioned in the ancient texts the *Kama Sutra* (from roughly 400 BC) and my personal fave, *The Joy of Sex* (from a forgotten time when people still had pubes—1972).

BDSM players come in all shapes and sizes. You can be 5 feet tall, 100 pounds soaking wet and be the most awesome Dom on the planet. Conversely, you can be a big, strapping male corporate executive who likes wearing frilly women's lingerie and giving pedicures. In BDSM, you are free to be you . . . and me! However, if you've been looking at magazines or on the 'net, you've likely seen perfect looking models carrying out BDSM scenarios. In real life, there are plenty of regular, even terribly ugly (kidding) people doing this stuff.

When I first started working at a dungeon, one of the employers suggested I dye my hair blonde to attract more clientele. I then suggested that while plenty of clients might want to spank Sandra Dee, maybe a brunette with a round ass and perky tits might do. Shockingly, I was right. The BDSM community is diverse and everyone's tastes are different. Haters gon' hate, but there is plenty of love for everyone, so embrace who you are. It's really all about attitude and confidence. However, there are some basic "types" of which you should be familiar.

Roles You Can Play in BDSM

Tops—The partners who carry out the activities. They do a lot of work. (A general term that encompasses both sadists and Doms.)

bottoms—The recipients of the activities. They get to lie around a lot. (Again, a general term encompassing both subs and masochists.)

Dominants—Those who like to dominate. (Think James Spader in *Secretary* . . . boing!)

submissives—Those who like to submit. (They don't even get capitalization! That's how submissive they are!) Someone once said to me, "A submissive gets off on getting their partner off." This is true, though I'd like to think subs get off, too. (And they should, especially if they've been good.)

Sadists—Those who enjoy inflicting pain. (Think Marquis de Sade who was such a sadistic bastard that the words *sadism* and *sadist* are derived from his name.) Side note: The majority of sadists are not bastards at all. For the most part, they inflict pain for erotic gratification on masochists (see below) who *gain* erotic gratification from said pain.

masochists—Those who enjoy pain. (The term is named after Leopold von Sacher-Masoch whose novel *Venus in Furs* explores a sadomasochistic relationship.) Important point: Masochists enjoy pain in a safe, consensual, erotic environment, so don't think you can just walk up to one on the street and roundhouse kick him in the nuts. He will likely kick you back—or have you arrested.

Mistress—A term for a female Dom.

Master—A term for a male Dom.

Mommy—A Mistress who acts "maternally."

Daddy—A Dom who acts "paternally." (Can be male or female.)

Perv—While some might view this as a derogatory term, as "one who is perverted" or whose sexual tastes deviate from the norm, throughout the book I will use it as a term of endearment, mostly for my friends who are pervs.

Risk-Aware Consensual Kink (RACK, also **Risk-Accepted Consensual Kink)**—This acronym is used to describe a view that is generally permissive of certain risky sexual behaviors, as long as the participants are fully aware of the risks. This differs from the safe, sane, and consensual mode in that it recognizes that both partners are informed of the risks involved in the proposed activity.

Prick—(**PRICK,** also **Personal Responsibility, Informed Consensual Kink**) is yet another term for BDSM activities, one that emphasizes taking responsibility for one's own actions, much like RACK above.

Switch—A switch is someone who participates in BDSM activities sometimes as a top and other times as a bottom.

For example . . .

During my first week as a pro sub, I was shocked when mid-session a client named "Pete" said to me, "I'm a switch. Do you know what that means?" Without waiting for an answer, he continued, "I see Mistresses and submissives. The Mistresses here like to fuck my ass with dildos. Would you do that for me?"

"Sure," I agreed, and then quickly thought, *WHAT am I doing?* But a deal's a deal and before I had to time to think of a way out, he'd laid out three dildos, draped in condoms and ready to go. The largest of the three dildos was . . . like no human penis on Earth. It was *monstrous*. But I did eventually fuck him with all three dildos while he yelled, "Fuck me! Fuck me!" The giant dildo slid in just as easily as the small one. It was like watching a sword swallower at work. (Not sure if this was legal and am guessing it wasn't, but I was young and naive and the rules were never spelled out for me so . . . Don't show up at your local dungeon looking for someone to fuck you in the ass with dildos.) Legality aside, it made Pete come buckets!

Since then, I've always had a special place in my heart for those who switch. A couple years ago, I even found *myself* switching from my generally submissive nature to that of a domineering tyrant. When I met a powerful, gorgeous man who happened to have a go-go boot fetish (the result of watching Nancy Sinatra dance on TV during his formative years), I was more than happy to let him bend down and kiss my pink, pleather boots. Not only did I love the experience, but this gentleman also explained fetishes better than any sexologist I've ever met:

"Some people think I'm a pervert because I like boots," he said (in an incredibly sexy British accent). "Those people didn't see Nancy Sinatra on TV that day."

Becoming an Endor-Fan!

Sometimes it's hard to get "high on life." Personally, I have been "high on life" for forty years and it's never really done the trick. Luckily, we have something called endorphins of which I am an endor-fan!

As mentioned previously, I am not a sexologist nor am I a doctor. The closest I've ever come to understanding the workings of the human body came from doing a magazine interview with Slim Goodbody, the 1970s "superhero of health" who wore a disturbing organ-painted unitard and used to do songs and dances about hormones and vital organs on Saturday morning TV. In one episode I'll never forget, he talked about endorphins.

Endorphins are amazing little fuckers—a group of hormones secreted within the brain and nervous system that have a number of physiological functions. They are peptides that activate the body's opiate receptors, causing an analgesic effect. (Meaning endorphins activate our body's natural painkillers.)

Why am I telling you all this? Because while it's easy for an outsider or someone who is new to BDSM to understand why being Dominant rocks (lots of power and control plus cool latex outfits and boots), many are perplexed by submissives—and especially by masochists. And while there is still plenty of research to be done on the subject, one thing is certain: when your ass gets spanked or flogged or caned, endorphins are released. And for some, it feels awesome. This is why some people enjoy pain: because a good ass spanking is certainly easier to get than Percocet.

Chains, Whips, and Cuffs

Endorphins are one of the many reasons I caution against engaging in play while wasted (especially on anything that might make the sub insensitive to pain, such as heroin—which you shouldn't do anyway, so as to avoid dying). BDSM is like its own drug.

However, I see nothing wrong with a little beer, wine, or even weed (not that I would *ever* advocate the use of an illegal substance!). In fact, as both a beer enthusiast and a submissive, there have been a couple of times where I've been tied up and have had to beg for a sip of frothy beer from my play partner. And I can tell you with certainty that a single sip of even the cheapest domestic beer tastes *great* under these circumstances.

Types of BDSM Relationships

Now what happens when you get all these endorphins and folks—the Tops and bottoms, sadists and masochists, corporate execs in lingerie, Lilliputians in PVC, and switches—together? Magic, that's what! That, and complicated relationships, for which there are innumerable definitions and titles. Attempting to list each variance would be like reciting the contents of the produce aisle at Whole Foods.

Since you are reading a BDSM starter book, I'm guessing you and your partner are just beginning to play in the bedroom. This is what is commonly known as Bedroom D/s. It takes place during a set time frame, involves sensual Dominance and submission, and usually coincides with sex. There is no power exchange outside of the bedroom (or whatever room you choose to make nookie in). So, say your girlfriend occasionally enjoys being tied up and spanked before *or* while getting fucked—that in no way means you have the right to demand she hand you the remote without at least saying please.

There is also a chance you got this starter book because you are single and want to get involved in BDSM. In that case, it's a good idea to know what types of relationships and scenarios are out there so you don't suddenly find yourself sealed away in an inaccessible castle a la *120 Days of Sodom.*

While researching this book, I held a "conference" at Mr. Hall's apartment wherein I discussed BDSM with Mr. Hall and two of the hottest women on the planet: burlesque performers "Amanda Whip" and "Scooter Pie." Both women have great expertise in BDSM. Amanda has worked as a pro Dom for a several years and is generally a kinky lesbian with a great imagination. (*And* she recently posed for a racy *Penthouse* pictorial that accompanied a story I wrote for them.) Scooter Pie is also a kinky self-professed slut who has worked as a pro Dom off and on for years. Plus, she's something of a sexpert, given she worked at the sex toy superstore Babeland for three years.

Check it out!

Much like this book, Babeland celebrates "the simple truth that sexually healthy people make the world a happier place." If you are looking for cool sex toys and information on all things carnal, check out their website http://www.babeland.com. It's where a friend bought me my first vibrator (a rabbit), which I eventually had to throw out because I wasn't getting any writing done.

I thought, since I have been mostly submissive, it would be a good idea to discuss BDSM with this kooky panel, who are all far more dominant than me. (I also secretly hoped our conference would end in an orgy, which it didn't because I had to go home and work on this goddamned book.)

The first question I put out to the panel of sexperts was: "Why not just fuck? Why try BDSM?"

"Why eat only for nutrition?" Amanda asked in response.

One of many good points made that night. If sex is like strawberries, BDSM is chocolate-covered strawberries.

I also asked them what the most misunderstood things about BDSM are.

"People think anyone who is into it is just a drug-addicted whore," Amanda answered succinctly.

Anyone who's been part of a BDSM scene knows this isn't the case. When doing it professionally, I did have some coworkers with substance abuse problems (half the world has them), but the majority of my coworkers were well-educated women who more often than not had their shit together and were working toward advanced degrees (albeit in totally unusable fields of study). Our clients were, for the most part, decent people. Most of them looked like they belonged in what we called the "vanilla world." That's one thing about BDSM—you never know who's into it.

After a recent bondage story of mine was published in *Penthouse*, I got a Facebook message from a guy I'd been on the swim team with as a teenager and hadn't heard from in years. It started: "Just read your story in *Penthouse*! Guess you never know who you're getting in the water with! Great work!"

He was right on the money: You never know who you're getting in the water with. Some of the most normal people I've dated (there haven't been many) have had some of the weirdest kinks, whereas many of the freaks I've dated have been completely vanilla in the sack.

Scooter thought the greatest misconception regarding BDSM is that "people think it's all about pain. They don't get the nuances."

As the acronym suggests it *isn't* all about pain, but also about Dominance and submission. (This is why it's sometimes just referred to as D/s, but for the sake of consistency, I use the term "BDSM" throughout.) So if BDSM isn't all about pain, *what* is it about? In a word: power. And human beings value power more than sex. If we didn't, anytime there was a squabble about territory or food, we'd just fuck like bonobo chimpanzees, for who sex functions in conflict appeasement. (They truly get the slogan "Make Love, Not War." I hope to be reincarnated as one.)

So then what are the power dynamics of BDSM? Together, we four pervs (Amanda, Scooter, Mr. Hall, and I) discussed the nuances along with the many types of BDSM relationships and several other topics to be covered later. Note that these relationships are not limited by gender or sexual identity. The BDSM community is a welcoming one, where all that's required to be a part of it is a willingness to identify with it. But in terms of relationships and scenarios, there are many varieties out there. During our discussion, we made an effort to identify the very basics.

The Four Basic BDSM Food Groups

"Bedroom D/s" or **"Vanilla"**—Don't want to be redundant, but again, this is kind of like "doing it" with a little kink. Maybe sometimes you drip hot wax on your partner or stick a butt plug in his ass while you are fucking him. Maybe you even call your lover a bitch or a slut while you're fucking her, quite possibly while she has a butt plug in her ass or is wearing a blindfold or crotchless panties or even a Nixon mask or some other zany costume. *Maybe* you even call your lover a cum-guzzling, tea-bagging whore while she is wearing said Nixon mask and crotchless panties and has a butt plug in her ass. Maybe *you* have a butt plug in *your* ass—a vibrating one at that, and your lover is wearing a nun's habit and a Nixon mask and crotchless panties and you are both calling each other cum-guzzling slut-bag whores while fucking. Point is "vanilla" means you don't have the right to call each other bitches, sluts, or cum-guzzling, tea-bagging whores at a dinner party. You leave that shit in the bedroom.

"Casual Play"—It's hardly fair to even call this a "relationship," but casual play is when two people get together during a negotiated play time and do a "scene." Maybe it only happens once. Maybe it happens at a party. Maybe there is no sex involved. Example: A friend of mine just "casually" got together with another friend and gave her a "session" for her birthday. He spanked and flogged her, got her endorphins going, and then the two hugged and ate cake. This type of BDSM play is like wearing jeans to work: very relaxing.

"Can I Just Have a Sandwich?"—This type of relationship is normally dubbed a Total Power Exchange (TPE) or sometimes it's simply called 24/7. Both terms refer to a relationship where the Dom or owner has complete authority and influence over the submissive's life and makes the majority of decisions. In most TPE relationships, the partners play

at anytime and in anyplace.
A 24/7 lifestyle is very
demanding and will suck
up most of your time and
emotional energy, which is
why I have renamed it "Can I
Just Have a Sandwich?" The
name is in honor of my friend,
Mr. Hall, who was in a 24/7
relationship a few years back.

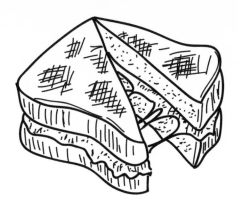

"Never again!" he exclaimed. "I got so tired of being the Master all the
time and just wanted to have a sandwich, you know. I'd be filling up
her dog bowl with water and just thinking, 'Can't I just relax and have a
fucking sandwich?' "

"Yeah," Amanda Whip agreed. "Sometimes you just wanna have a
sandwich on a table and not her back."

And there you have it. A total power exchange is a lot of work. You
might have to fill up your lover's dog bowl thrice daily while he or she
pretends to be your pet and you might not get to eat a sandwich off of a
table for several years. Just be prepared.

"Paid Sessions"—Maybe I'll catch flak for including this as a
"relationship" category, but in the BDSM world, paid sessions are
common. Many people can't find partners or lovers who are willing to
fulfill their kinks, so they go to professionals. Because I'm always doing
"research," I often asked my clients at the dungeon why they came to me.
One particularly heavy client (*heavy* meaning he was into tons of caning
and other painful corporeal scenes) told me, "My wife doesn't get it. She
thinks blowjobs are kinky. If she knew what I was *really* into, she'd leave
me." Hence paid sessions supply something for which there is a great
demand: understanding eroticism without judgment.

On with the Show!

(The "nuts" and bolts and fun stuff . . .)

As promised, we'll now get to some actual lessons. In the next few sections, we'll discuss techniques, equipment, outfits, and even home décor! You'll also learn how to flog, tie up, and humiliate your loved one. If you are submissive, you will get an idea of how some of these things feel, but mostly you can just be a lazy ass and hand this book to your lover. (Kidding again!)

I've often said the difference between sadists and masochists is that masochists are just lazy, but this is only partly true—especially if you are a pushy bottom who likes to dictate how everything goes down. This is oft referred to as "topping from the bottom."

When first hired at the dungeon, a Dominatrix said to me, "As a submissive, you have more power than you know. *You* control the session." In many ways, this is true. As both Voltaire and the Spiderman movie pointed out, "With great power comes great responsibility." To make another superhero analogy, if your partner has a thigh-high stocking fetish and you think of your lover as Superman, the stockings you wear are Kryptonite.

As a sub, you also have the power to stop a session at anytime by using your safe word. Don't be afraid to use it. Just as there are masterful Doms, there are also masterful submissives. Knowing what you want and learning how to communicate this are crucial to mastering the art of submission. That's why we are going to start with language.

During "normal" sex (i.e., nothing involving whips, ropes, chains, wax, role-play, or any of the other stuff described herein), a lot of people fuck in total silence. Sometimes they fuck to smooth jazz or rock 'n' roll.

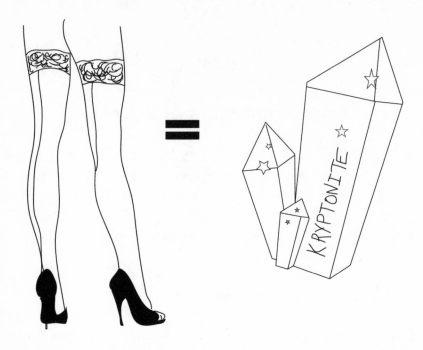

Point is, they don't have to talk all that much. Maybe one partner has to say "Get a condom!" or "Pass me the lube!" But intercourse tends to be relatively simple. In BDSM there is a lot to discuss, but if you are new to the scene, finding the right vocabulary for expressing your wants and needs can be a daunting task. Luckily, I am here to guide you . . .

Talk Dirty to Me!

(It's not just a bitchin' Poison song . . .)

I've read plenty of books about sex. (Shocking, I know.) And many of these books advocate the use of "dirty talk." Though I'm a good talker, I *used* to fail miserably when it came to dirty talk. Then, while attending an orgy (one of many I went to for "research" while working as a columnist), I met a man who called himself the Headmaster. He suggested that for my next column, I enroll in his S&M academy, the Princess Reform School, which I mentioned earlier.

Unlike other reform schools, which are devoted to making bad students good, Princess Reform School is dedicated to making good students *bad*. Before our first lesson, the Headmaster requested I list and rank my "problem areas." Was I too modest, too bratty, or too haughty? Perhaps I was insufficiently skilled in erotic service? The ranking would help determine emphasis in my lesson. Despite the fact that I'd gotten naked in a good 50 percent of my columns, I was still a shrinking violet when it came to public nudity, so modesty ranked high. Shyness while engaging in dirty talk, sexual laziness, and a general insolence toward authority also made the top of the list.

The Headmaster surveyed my list and then gave me my first homework assignment. Homework? I shuddered at the thought, but thankfully PRS homework didn't involve memorizing dates or learning times tables. Instead it entailed going to a Barnes & Noble wearing a miniskirt *sans panties*. Once there I was to peruse a wealth of information found in two books he highly recommended—*Erotic Surrender: The Sensual Joys of Female Submission* by Claudia Varrin and *Talk Dirty to Me: An Intimate Philosophy of Sex* by Sallie Tisdale.

Of course, it was the windiest day of the year, so on the way there, I shocked an entire double-decker bus full of tourists by inadvertently exposing my hairless clam. But once there, I found the required reading, slid onto a wooden chair (praying a splinter wouldn't pierce my labia), and learned quite a bit about dirty talk.

One of the most important techniques was that of "call and response." It makes dirty talk *so* much easier. Basically, the Dom asks you a question and you repeat the question in your response. (If you are the Dom, you actually have to think of the question, so it's a bit tougher.)

How to Train Your Filthy Mouth

Example #1

Dom: Do you want me to tie you to the bed and fuck the shit out of you with my big fat cock?

sub: Yes, I want you to tie me to the bed and fuck the shit out of me with your big fat cock!

Dom: Say "please, Sir."

sub: Please, Sir!

See? Doesn't take a whole lot of thought.

So as not to be sexist, let's give an example of how a female Dom might use this technique with a male. (And then we'll stop. I would love to go through the litany of every sexual variation, but this is an instructional guide, not some cheap porno mag!)

How to Train Your Filthy Mouth

Example #2

Dom: Do you wanna suck my 12-inch strap-on, you trashy pussy bottom boy?

sub: Yes, Mistress! I wanna suck your 12-inch strap-on please!

Easy enough. Note that in BDSM, manners are important. Always say "please" and "thank you" and find out what your Dom likes to be called beforehand. As a professional sub, I found that some Doms preferred "Master" while others preferred "Sir" or "Lord." Weirdly, I always liked using "Lord," possibly because I've read too much Tolkien or attended far too many Renaissance Faires.

Aside from "call and response," there are plenty of other ways to ease into dirty talk. Try to avoid clinical words like *vagina* and *penis*. (I am forty and the word *penis* still makes me laugh.) Go instead for porn classics like *cock* and *pussy*. Or throw a little Tantric Sex in the mix and tell him you want every inch of his erect lingam. (Sanskrit for penis.) As someone who discovered the joys of Tantric Sex after years of BDSM play, I found that both have a lot in common in that they utilize sexual arousal to reach altered states of awareness. Both also take planning and time, though I can hardly think of time better spent.

Getting back to dirty talk, flattery, again, is a great policy. Tell your lover she has perfect tits and I guarantee her vertical smile will shine. And unless your lover likes to be verbally humiliated (we're getting to that next), tell him he's got a great cock.

And for the love of God, if you are going to sext, make sure you are sexting to the intended recipient—unless you want your roommate and everyone else in the pub to know that later you'd like your lover to blindfold, cuff, cane, and fuck you. (Not that I speak from experience or anything . . .)

Another powerful tool in BDSM is silence. The best session I ever had was with a gentleman who, while in town on business, visited the "counseling center" for a session. He said only a few sentences to me over the course of an hour. "Bend over the horse," "Are you wet?" and "Are you going to come?" were among them. Let's just say I answered the final question in the affirmative.

The man knew how to give a good spanking and he was *a true gentleman*. No filthy tighty-whities on this one. He was well-groomed, sharply dressed, manicured, and clean. As mentioned previously, manners are important in BDSM, not just when speaking, but when dressing and preparing for a session. And since we're going there . . .

> # A note on hygiene:
>
> It's a relatively simple concept that doesn't require its own chapter or even its own paragraph.
>
> *Please wash your ass.*

Verbal Humiliation

Since we're talking about talk, I figured we'd just jump ahead to verbal humiliation! Most BDSM guidebooks start with whipping, spanking, or bondage, but we're just gonna get crazy here. Because the mental component of BDSM is as important as the physical, learning to creatively humiliate your submissive is crucial.

Due to my awkward, clumsy nature, I am *great* at humiliating myself and have never had to *ask* for humiliation or hire a professional to help with the task. I'm quite dumbass enough as it is, thank you. However, while I'm great at humiliating myself, I am terrible at humiliating others. Most of my life is spent gingerly trying to protect the fragile human ego. I am just that sensitive.

Over-Acting

Some of my favorite times at the dungeon were with pro Doms whose clients requested a submissive join in their session. These events were comical more often than not. One evening, Anastasia, a Russian Dom with sandy blond hair and a body like a Bond Girl, requested my presence midway through a session with her client "Joseph." Anastasia intimidated the shit out of me. If we were on Themyscira, she was Wonder Woman (albeit blond and Russian). I had no idea what to expect, but when we got to the door, she started giggling. I had never seen her laugh before.

"You gonna love this," she said, busting open the door.

Joseph looked to be in his early fifties, slender with graying hair. He wore only a pair of blue manties. His wrists were chained to two posts above his head and his ankles were tied to two posts on the floor. The entire room reeked of pot smoke. It was like Spicoli's van. The radio was tuned to classic rock. A Steely Dan song played.

"Do you know VOT this FUCKING HIPPIE VOS doing in here before the session even STARTED?" Anastasia bellowed. Her accent's severity had doubled since we entered the room. She sounded like Dracula meets Natasha Fatale.

"No, Mistress," I said.

"He VOS SMOKING POT!" At this, she gave his ass a smack with her hand.

She spent the next the next half-hour berating Joseph for being a hippie (with terrible taste in music) while also taunting him that he wasn't allowed to touch my half-naked body while she got to caress it all she wanted. She was a great "over-actress" and I realized then that BDSM is often a magical land of make-believe.

Another Use for "Call and Reponse"

I've found that "call and response" also works with verbal humiliation, sometimes in the form of forced flattery or forced admission of ownership. One Master repeatedly smacked my breasts with a riding crop while asking me, "Whose breasts are these?"

"They're *yours*, Sir," I responded, which was, of course, the correct answer.

Sometimes, a Dom would point to his small penis and say, "How do you like this massive cock?"

And I would say, "It's very impressive, Sir."

More from the Sexperts

While great at (even insincere) flattery, my humiliation skills are weak. Luckily, Mr. Hall, Scooter, and Amanda have no problem being complete assholes. (In safe, sane, consensual settings, of course.) And they were happy to share tips.

"How do you humiliate someone?" I asked Amanda.

"How do you *not*?" she retorted, in essence, humiliating me. "How could stuff not come into your head about how stupid and pathetic people are?"

Good point.

"Usually," Amanda added, "I just talk to subs about how they are perverts and everyone knows that all they think about is sex. You can also criticize his features. If they are paying clients, I make fun of them for paying. I'll say, 'You old, fat, hairy piece of shit! You have to come in here and pay me to beat your ass because no one else will!' They love that."

Mr. Hall added that this scenario could be played out between a husband and wife. The wife could pretend to be a Dominatrix who the husband is paying. She could then say, "You old, fat, hairy piece of shit! I bet while you're paying me, your wife is fucking someone else!"

Scooter had an interesting take on humiliation, in that her preferred method is not to use cruelty, but to get her partners (or more likely, clients) to do things to amuse her just because she's making them do them. (Cheerleading cheers, silly costumes, and animal noises were all mentioned). "The goal for me here is more about humor than arousal, although I do find laughing very sexy," she added.

> One of the great things about BDSM play is that it is *play*.
> Things don't have to make complete sense.

Mr. Hall then shared, "When my girlfriend and I are doing a scene, she is always worried the neighbors are gonna hear, so I make her scream, 'I'm a dirty whore and I love my Master's cock in my ass!' I make her repeat it until she comes."

"Have the neighbors ever complained?" I asked.

"No, but it drives her wild." Turns out, his ladylove is actually an exhibitionist and he found her "trigger."

Repetition

When it comes to humiliation, repetition is key. Usually there is one phrase or sentence that will make a sub explode with pleasure. One of the "rooms" at the dungeon where I worked was decorated like a schoolroom, only it was filled with whips and chains and books that no one ever read along with a desk, which people never sat at unless they were tied to it. It wasn't unusual to walk into the "schoolroom" and find that someone had scrawled "I will not be a slut" about a hundred times on the chalkboard.

Make sure you pre-negotiate what type of humiliation your sub prefers.

Amanda, Mr. Hall, and Scooter all agreed that there are certain trigger words that just do it for some subs. Sometimes these are un-PC phrases that rational adults wouldn't use in everyday interactions, like "dirty little faggot."
While certain racial and ethnic slurs might give some dudes raging boners, other dudes might be traumatized for life just hearing them. While one woman might enjoy having her small breasts criticized, another might find this type of derision is too much.
You want your partner to get off, not spend years in therapy.

During my time at the dungeon, I was called many things, but namely a whore, a slut, and a bitch. These were all pretty accurate actually! In fact, when called a "bitch" (even outside of the dungeon), I have always responded with "thank you," since the word is derived from an Old Norse term for female canine. And if you've ever watched a nature special on female wolves or been lucky enough to see one in nature, you know these bitches have great instincts and are extremely intelligent, good caregivers, incredibly loyal, curious, and beautiful!

Which is why this conversation happens so often:

Dom: You are an insolent bitch!

Me: Thank you, Sir!

While "bitch," "slut," and "whore" are great, get creative! My panel of experts all suggested that the list of things one can say to joyfully humiliate his or her loved one or play partner is endless.

Amanda was full of suggestions. "You can make fun of him for having a small penis *even if he has a large penis,* for being fat *even if he's skinny,* for being weak with no muscles, wearing ugly shoes, you know . . . poor taste in general."

Mr. Hall added, "You can also chide her for being a slut or even a cock-crazed dirty slut or for being a pussy-worshipping faggot *even though this makes no sense.* 'Limp dick' works, but not 'dry pussy.' I don't know why . . ."

"You could make fun of her for being such a slut, she has a soaking pussy," I suggested.

"Exactly."

I was already getting the hang of it.

Your Turn!

What have you always wanted your partner to say to you in bed? And what do you hope he or she *never* says? List these on the lines below— and be honest! If hearing a specific word is a complete turn off, it's important to let your partner know ahead of time. Otherwise things will go downhill—fast.

These humiliating words get me hot.	If you say these words, you will have to pay for my twice-weekly therapy.

Physical Humiliation

Physical humiliation is a whole other ball game, one where parameters should also be set ahead of time. If you are a Dom, don't just sneak up on your sub and shove a butt plug in his or her ass. Make sure he or she *wants* that butt plug (or candle or set of anal beads or whatever else gets inserted into asses nowadays) *in* his or her ass first.

In my experience, body worship is one of the most common forms of physical humiliation. While doing sessions at the Chelsea with Annie, she would often lead me by a leash to our Master's feet, on my hands and knees, blindfolded, cuffed, and wearing little else. She would then say, "Caress your Master's body," and I would (usually while she caressed me). Sometimes she would tell me to kiss my Master's feet and, if I wasn't doing it "properly," she would tell me to use my tongue (a verbal/physical combo!).

As with verbal humiliation, the varieties of physically humiliating acts a Dom can command are endless. A few I experienced at the dungeon were forced masturbation, having to ask if I were allowed to have an orgasm during said forced masturbation, being spat on, being slapped, being used as a footstool, and so on. With boyfriends and lovers, the physical humiliation has been more sexual in nature—namely being ejaculated on. (Note: When they are aiming for the face, keep your eyes closed or have plenty of Visine handy.)

On one rare occasion when I was hired for a Dom session, *I* did the humiliating, dragging a timid gentleman out into the reception area on a leash so the other Mistresses could see his raging boner. I told him if he didn't go with me, I would pee all over his face. (When we got back to the room, I then made him jack off in his own hand.) Another time, I applied a client's makeup and dressed him in the beautiful evening gown that he'd brought with him. Interestingly enough, he brought a matching gown for me, which I put on. Once we were all dressed up with nowhere to go, he simply wanted to be called a "pretty girl." (He actually was quite pretty. I thought he looked better in the gown than I did.)

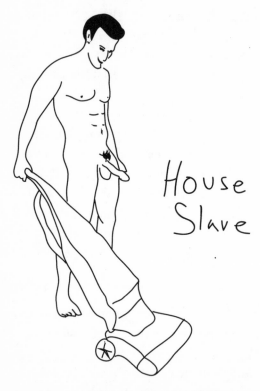

House Slave

At the dungeon we had plenty of "house slaves." These were dudes who ran errands and acted as maids for us at no fee as long as we humiliated them. It wasn't unusual to arrive at work to find one such slave vacuuming naked. Sometimes we made them run out and get us lunch (their treat), ChapStick®, Dr. Scholl®'s insoles, moisturizer, and anything else we wanted. Occasionally the Mistresses wrote "bitch" on both sides of the house slave's hands so he would be publicly humiliated upon paying. If you are a slob, getting your own house slave isn't such a bad idea.

A great deal of BDSM play could be considered physical humiliation, whether it's erotic objectification (using your sub's back as a table upon which you eat the aforementioned sandwich), making them perform a spirited cheer in your honor, or simply jizzing on your sub's face. The only real limit is your imagination, boundaries, and budget. (Not everyone can afford a new evening gown!)

Your Turn!

What have you always wanted your partner to do to you in bed?
And what do you hope he or she *never* does? List these on the lines
below—and, again, be honest! If being touched, grabbed, or prodded
in a certain area will make you flip shit, your partner needs to know.
This will prevent many black eyes and swift kicks to the boys (or,
perhaps, girls).

These forms of physical humiliation give me a woody/clit boner.	Doing any of these will just piss me off.

Spanking

Since we're now speaking of budgetary restrictions, let's talk about spanking. It really is the "backbone" of BDSM—relatively simple to perform and, in these rough financial times, it's economical, too. The only tools required are a hand and an ass.

I say "relatively" simple because while "hard" and "soft" might seem like the only variances, there are many ways to spank your special someone.

Warning!

Though earlier I encouraged doing extra research on BDSM, I am now going to *discourage* you from researching spanking on the Internet where you will invariably happen upon creepy blogs penned by over-religious, zealot douche bags wherein they give instructions on spanking children *and* wives as a form of punishment. (This makes me shudder.) These blogs are gross and sad—gross for the obvious reasons and sad because the abused often become abusers themselves.

At the dungeon, the clients I considered the "heaviest" (the men I would deem actual sadists) had almost always suffered abuse during childhood. These were individuals who had been frequently spanked to a point of bruises and tears and then later eroticized the horrors of their childhood to deal with them. Luckily, they found an outlet at the dungeon for the things that haunted them the most.

This is where I see sex workers as being an invaluable part of the community. Not everyone can express this stuff to a doctor or psychiatrist. I am not a shrink, but I knew this stuff about my former clients because they would tell me. Maybe these clients didn't actually go to shrinks. Maybe they just came to me because, for about the same cost as a shrink, I got half naked, listened to them talk, *and* let them spank me.

Whatever the case, I cannot speak for all sadists, and this was not always the case, but I saw too many examples to count. One regular client of mine had, in his youth, been forced to watch his mother beat his little sister with a wooden hairbrush. The mother wouldn't stop until his sister cried. His solution? Pay me to wear a schoolgirl costume and spank me with a wooden hairbrush until I "cried." I feel like this man should have been able to sue his parents for all the money he spent at the dungeon trying to cope.

Sorry for the psychoanalytic digression, but I just want it to be extra crystal clear: The kind of spanking we are talking about in this chapter is NOT any form of domestic discipline. It has absolutely nothing to do with minors or with "teaching" your wife a "lesson." We are talking about *erotic* spanking, namely sensual, good times. (And if you did have a crap childhood, the possible side bonus of a cathartic, emotional release.)

So why, on an erotic level, would anybody want to spank anybody else?

There are many reasons. The first and most obvious is to repeatedly touch and caress the attractive ass of your lover. Secondly, being the "spanker" gives you a sense of control and power. Thirdly, knowing the "spankee" is getting aroused, that he is popping wood or that she is getting wet from your spanking, is beyond exciting. If you are both *sexual* BDSM partners, there is a very good chance the spanking will lead to smokin' sex. In fact, if you're a multi-tasker, you can *continue* the spanking during intercourse. It's not always just a warm-up exercise.

Now, why would anybody want to be the spankee?

We already covered endorphins (endor-fun!), but physical sensation is just half of it. Let's start with the physical: The ass is indeed an erogenous zone, but it's one that is usually covered in a layer of fat, which is why we're not all walking around having ass-gasms constantly. The ass requires a little something more—namely squeezing, spanking, and massaging. Is there anything better than an ass massage? I think not. The only *bad* thing about ass massages is that they generally don't last more than two minutes. So a spanking can feel amazing—the warmth of a hand caressing your ass, the expectation of when that hand is going to land on your ass, and the rush of pleasure and pain that ultimately comes from that hand spanking your ass. It can give you a high, almost like a "runner's high" without the misery of running.

But being the spankee has yet an even greater appeal factor: Attention! Getting spanked means getting a lot of *attention,* and who doesn't love attention? (Okay, some people, but certainly not this Leo author.) Feeling that one's ass is coveted and desired and that *you* are coveted and desired is thrilling. Knowing that the higher you thrust your bottom in the air, the more excited your partner gets, feels *good.*

If you are new to spanking, as the spanker or the spankee, there are some things you might want to consider. Check out the handy list of suggestions.

Things to Consider About Your Bootylicious Adventure

The Noise Factor. There is *no silencer* for a hand on an ass. Do you have roommates? Nosy neighbors? Married with screaming little bastards? Before you cover your walls in egg cartons for sound insulation, consider a few options:

First, make sure your shithead roommates aren't home, and if you've got kids, get a babysitter to watch your screaming little bastards and find a room! Secondly, get some music going. You will find a lot of "sex manuals" wherein they recommend specific playlists for fucking. Out of curiosity, I polled my three thousand Facebook friends on what exactly they like to make nookie to and you will find the hilarious, somewhat disturbing results at the end of this chapter.

However, I am not going to tell you what to fuck or spank to (Portishead gets old fast . . .) but I will tell you this: Studies have shown that like sex, music we like makes dopamine go to the brain and do a sexy dance.

What the hell is dopamine? An alternative rock quartet from Caerphilly, Wales? Yes, but it is also a neurotransmitter and given it kind of has the word "dope" in it, you know it's gonna be good. Basically, dopamine modulates the brain's ability to perceive reward reinforcement. So, the pleasure sensation that the brain gets when dopamine levels are elevated creates the motivation for us to proactively perform actions that are indispensable to our species' survival (like fucking). Hence, when a person comes he or she is flooded with this awesome and meddlesome neurotransmitter and listening to music we dig releases just a tiny bit of it, kind of like a "tease."

Long story short, play music when you are spanking your partner and he or she will be sure to thrust his or her ass that much higher in the sky. It will also drown out the sound of hand on ass. What to play? *Who cares!* Presumably you are with your partner or lover because he or she have a similar taste in music as you do. Personally, I cannot get a clit boner if my partner doesn't appreciate Pink Floyd or Zeppelin the way I do. If I went home with a man and he put on Nickelback, I would go flaccid and question the very foundation of my existence.

But I do have one tiny suggestion: Get a record player. Nothing fancy, just some crappy thing you find at a flea market. Collecting old, weird records with your partner and knowing that you will both fuck or spank or masturbate to *Tiny Tim's Christmas Album* later is a bonding experience. So is "getting up" to "flip the record." Flipping the record practically predates putting on a condom as one of those awkward but necessary moves that, thanks to the ingenuity of the human race, allows us to experience a dopamine rush without the result of procreation.

Are your hands cold and clammy? There is only one thing worse than a limp handshake and that is cold, clammy hands spanking your ass! Make certain, if you are the spanker, that you warm up your hands before going to town on your sub's bottom.

Start *slowly*. Don't just lift your hand all the way in the air and bring it down with a thud. Take your time. For this chapter, I again consulted Mr. Hall, who loves to spank. He had this to say:

> "As in all BDSM play, I start by establishing the 'Red, Yellow, Green' safe words method, though with spanking this is rarely needed." (Here I might disagree with Mr. Hall because, even though the ass is the fattest part of my body and I have the pain threshold of an X-Men mutant, I have had to use safe words while being spanked a number of times.)

> "Mostly I can pick up on physical reactions to know when to slow down and when to wail on my happily weeping, willing, wanton woman," Mr. Hall added. "I've found the best position is me seated on the bed with my lover/sub either naked or with her pants pulled down, lying comfortably with ass positioned on the upper part of my right leg (not quite in the center of my lap). If she likes hair pulling, I'll grasp her hair with my left hand and give a few light spanks with my right hand, followed by some gentle rubbing. I repeat this a few times until I can see her near-begging for the 'real deal.' This either occurs via physical cues like her lifting and wiggling her butt, or a snide remark such as, 'Is this a fucking massage or are you are you going to beat my ass already?' Then the fun really begins!

> "With a tighter grasp on her hair, I'll deliver a few hard smacks on each cheek, check to see if she's responding well (a smile, once again, a wiggling butt), and if so I'll spank until her ass is red. Other than the aforementioned cues, how soft or hard is also dependent on how close I am to my partner and how long we've played. For example, if someone starts to pull away that could mean 'slow down' or it could mean 'pull my hair and spank me even harder for being a wimp.' "

Talk to your sub. Mr. Hall's last point is a good one. Playing with a familiar partner is much different than playing with a new one. As a Dom, *always* check in with your sub. You can do this by simply asking, "Do you want it harder?" Talk is important. Not just for setting boundaries, but for heating things up. Mr. Hall also suggested techniques such as, "You were forty minutes late and that means forty whacks on each cheek." You then have your sub count each one off. You can also whisper dirty things such as, "I know you love this, you dirty little pain slut. Stick that ass out and show me how much." And lastly (in the best of cases), "I love you so much and love that we love this." (whack, whack, whack!)

Incorporate Games. The sadist I mentioned earlier (schoolgirl getup, wooden hairbrush) loved to incorporate games into spanking. On one occasion, when Annie and I saw him on his birthday, he had us guess his age and for each year of his life we got one spanking, and for each year we were off we got two spankings. I remember thinking that he looked about 50. He was actually 51, so that made for a combined total of 53. Annie guessed 52, so she also got 53.

Change Positions. How to position your sub while spanking him or her is up to you. Many male Doms like the "over the lap" position because it means you are that much closer to their cock, which is presumably sporting a pants tent (if he is wearing pants at all). Personally, I always preferred standing up while getting spanked so that my partner could reach around and fondle my breasts. Kneeling on the floor (assuming it's not a cold linoleum floor) or on a bed or ottoman, stooped over with the hands on the floor below are also options, as is a simple over-the-knee position.

For example . . .

If you and your partner rent space in an actual dungeon or attend a party at a dungeon or sex club, you can get really creative with positions due to the wealth of equipment provided. At the dungeon, I was spanked numerous times while tied to a "medical" table with my feet in stirrups. Other times I was spanked while bent over a "horse" (a wooden inverted v-shaped sex toy that was originally used for torture). It was, while bent over one of these devices, that I had the "best session ever" mentioned earlier. My boss, the sex counselor/Dominatrix, gave me no other instructions but to bend over the horse and wait for the client. She also mentioned he wanted to spank me until I cried.

I remained bent over the horse as I heard the client close the door to the tiny room. His footsteps approached, but I remained perfectly still. He pressed gently against the wool fabric of my gray schoolgirl skirt and he moved his hands around, inspecting my "assets."

"You can stand up now," he said in the deep kind of voice that leaves not a dry vagina in the house. I stood up and turned to face him. To my surprise, his face was almost as lovely as his accent—high cheekbones, square jaw, black eyes, and brown hair that hung sloppily over his eyes. In contrast to his scruffy hair, his clothes were immaculate—a tailored navy suit and white shirt. But it was his black eyes that got me, the kind of eyes that don't reflect anything, so full of secrets they never sparkle.

"I am going to spank you," he said abruptly. "And, I want you to tell me when you are about to cry. It is very important that you be honest and that you really cry."

"Yes, Sir."

Moisture was already beginning to soak through my panties as he motioned for me to bend over the horse again. I bent over slowly, sticking my bottom out, inviting him, whereupon he began to spank me relentlessly. My ass stung and I closed my eyes, wondering if he could tell how wet I was. The spanking was unrelenting and he never slowed down. He didn't apologize. Didn't ask me if it was too hard. It *was* too hard, but for the first time ever, I wanted it *harder*. I stuck my ass out further, feeling as if I might die if he didn't rip my panties off and shove his cock into me. I couldn't see him, didn't dare turn around, but I knew he must be hard. He stood at a distance, didn't try to touch my pussy, didn't try to grab my breasts—all the usual stunts clients pulled.

I wanted to beg him, "*Please* fuck me. I can't take this," but I was afraid to make a sound. The room was completely quiet except for the sound of his hand spanking my ass. There was no role-play, no dialogue, nothing for me to say. I felt like I was on the brink of coming and he had barely touched me. Finally, I managed to stealthily reach my nimble fingers beneath my panties and sneakily polished my pearl.

"Are you going to come?" he asked. Guess I wasn't that sneaky.

"Yes," I gasped and did just that.

The spanking continued for about fifteen minutes when finally the pain became so intense that I thought I might cry. I was embarrassed to tell him, yet he instinctively knew.

"Are you going to cry?" he asked.

"Yes."

He leaned in order to watch me, but he continued spanking me as he did. I then did something that wasn't in the instructions, something submissives generally aren't supposed to do—I looked directly in his eyes. In that moment, all the secrets held in them fell away.

He took a break from spanking me to unzip his trousers and take out what I had correctly presumed was an erection. He then recommenced spanking me with one hand while he stroked his cock with his other. Soon thereafter, I started to cry. He reached out his finger and lightly touched my cheek for a millisecond, withdrawing it quickly as though he had just committed some horrible transgression. His breathing grew harder and in a few seconds, he came.

I was *soaked,* more turned on than I'd ever been in a session, and I think that says it all about the power of spanking. The mixed feelings of adoration and vulnerability one can experience as a spankee are overwhelming. And as the spanker, the feelings of power and control are intoxicating, especially when you have, in the past, been powerless or out of control.

Spanking Playlist

Now, as promised, the weirdest spanking/love making playlist ever compiled, as provided by my Facebook friends. One or two suggestions might actually do the trick, but realistically, many of these will cause immediate flaccidity. If you and your partner can get it on to any of these, you might actually be soul mates. Perhaps this is a true "soul mate litmus test."

Suggestions included . . .

"John Williams."

"A nice Irish reel."

"John Philip Sousa."

"Polka."

"The Ice Cream Truck Song."

"Faith No More."

"A guy in the corner playing Tchaikovsky's Sugarplum Fairy Theme on a xylophone."

"The music from one of those quarter amusement rides outside a supermarket!"

" 'I'm a Goofy Goober' from the Spongebob Movie soundtrack."

"Barbara Streisand singing Bowie's 'Life on Mars.' "

"Anything without lyrics. It's too distracting having someone singing in the room."

"Andre Williams or The Cramps."

"Barry White, the entire Miami Funk Series, Mahler, Dvorak, Wagner."

"Motley Crue and Danzig (both favorites of strippers the world over)."

My friend David mentioned that he had a girlfriend who could only come if Prince was on. He also shared, "I had a boss with a fertility problem (and what I imagined was an ever-doing-it problem). One day after lunch, he returned with a few Luther Vandross CDs. I said, 'That ought to do it!' He blushed—didn't know how obvious it was. Ten months later, he and his wife had a baby."

Chains, Whips, and Cuffs

Of my friends who participated in my poll and took it seriously, Otis Redding topped the list. Perhaps this is why Bill Clinton once said, "I remember when Otis Redding died; I didn't think I could go on."

I have a few rock star friends (I'm *that* cool) and one of them recently said to me, "I love it when I hear from fans and they tell me they lost their virginity to one of my songs." (If lucky, said fan loses it to an entire album, but that's beside the point.) Perhaps the subconscious goal of every musician is to increase our dopamine levels to the point where we are all fucking like rabbits.

At the dungeon, one great way to "time a session," which generally lasted an hour, was by playing a CD. (Because setting a stopwatch would have been kind of tacky.) A lot of Mistresses and subs opted for trip-hop, but personally, I played "groovy" stuff because groovy is how I like my sex, BDSM play, and pretty much everything else. T. Rex, The Zombies, The Beatles, and The Stones have never failed me.

Good sex and BDSM play should feel like a spell. Consider this as you spank your partner into a transcendent subspace.

Timing

A few words on timing:

Ironically, this will be the shortest section in the book. A good BDSM session *should* take time. Save quickies for drunken fucking in bar bathrooms. BDSM depends on a slow buildup. Rushing could lead to injuries and disappointment. Unless you are paying by the hour, give your session time. In Tantric Sex, it is suggested that partners hide their clocks or turn them towards the wall. I suggest the same for BDSM.

Speaking of a slow buildup, of sending your sub into the furthermost corners of transcendent subspace, vulnerability, and passion, let's now talk about flagellation. It's lots o' fun and people have been doing it for ages! (Seriously, it's been around since before the foundation of Rome . . .)

Flagellation

Flagellation or flogging is similar to spanking. It is defined as the act of methodically beating or whipping the human body. Unlike the more rudimentary and economical spanking, flagellation requires instruments. These include the cat o' nine tails, rods, switches, bullwhips, and canes. (Though usually I refer to using a cane as "caning.")

Historically, flogging was used as punishment on unwilling subjects. It still is in some places. Some religions practice self-flagellation (like certain constituents of the *Opus Dei* as seen in the Tom Hanks vehicle *The Da Vinci Code*). When flogging is submitted to willingly, it becomes part of BDSM.

Flog with Care!

One thing to remember when flogging that special someone: Careful where you do it! Places where you should *never* flog include the face, head, neck, fingers, toes, and over healing skin. Be aware of where the major organs are located, especially the kidneys, which are located toward the lower back and are therefore susceptible during flagellation—especially if your Dom lacks aim and coordination. If you think your Dom is coming a bit too close, say your safe word immediately.

In terms of where it's okay to flog lightly, the lower legs, arms, inner arms, breasts, upper shoulders, top of the ass, and genitals are acceptable. (Keep in mind that if your sub has breast implants, you might want to avoid flogging or whipping them entirely, as there is nothing sexy about a leaky implant.)

When it comes to heavy flogging, the buttocks are like air bags, able to take a whack delivered with momentum. (And, as mentioned previously, ass cheeks are an erogenous zone so have at 'em.) Other acceptable spots include the upper back on each side of the spine (leave that spine alone!), the thighs, and lower shoulders. Again, aim is crucial, so practice, practice, practice!

Mr. Hall shared a helpful tip: Use pillows. If your sub is lying face down and you are worried about accidentally flogging his or her most vulnerable parts, you can gently place a pillow over your partner's lower back and the backs of his or her knees. (You never want to flog joints.)

The Appropriate Equipment

When it comes to the wide range of flogging equipment out there, it's a good idea to familiarize yourself with how things are going to feel before using them on your partner.

For example . . .

My orientation at the dungeon involved Velocity Chyaldd giving me a tour through each room while explaining the equipment to me. We stood in the middle of the "medical room" and she looked me over like a bad girl in a Linda Blair "women in prison" movie. She had Bettie Page-style black hair and her lips were carefully painted red. Her waist was cinched together with an intricate ribbon-laced bustier. How would I ever get into such complicated clothing? At the time, I'd never owned any fetish gear. About the only thing I ever laced were my Converse high-tops and even those were sloppily undone half the time.

"Have you ever been suspended?" she asked.

"No," I answered, embarrassed by my lack of experience.

"You should try everything before you start. It'll make you more comfortable."

She motioned me toward the suspension bar.

I let her take my wrists and cuff them to the bar, which she raised using a nearby crank. Slowly I was elevated until my toes dangled off the ground. She tickled me lightly.

"Do you know what a cane feels like?"

"No." All I knew about canes is that they were used to severely punish graffitists and shoplifters in far-off lands.

"You don't ever *have* to agree to be caned. Personally, I can only take five or six at a time, but if you can take it, you'll get good tips."

I took a deep breath as my ass involuntarily clenched in expectation of the cane.

"I won't do it too hard," she promised. "Relax."

I tried to relax, but it was sort of like waiting for a shot at the doctor's office. I knew pain was on the horizon. She chose a cane from a basket of them and smacked my ass lightly with it. The sensation wasn't a thump; it was a sting, like instantaneous sunburn. I kind of liked it and pretty soon I was earning extra tips for my ability to "take a caning."

Canes are generally not used during light BDSM play. These bad boys, which are generally made of rattan, can cause excruciating pain (and pleasure) and are more for BDSM "heavy hitters." One of the things partners should discuss before a session is whether it's okay to leave marks on the sub's body. Canes sometimes break, but they can also break skin and leave marks. When caning your partner, you ideally want to strike him or her with the section of cane starting at the tip and extending perhaps 6 to 8 inches toward the handle.

Incorrectly striking your partner with only the tip can leave marks that take weeks to heal. It's a good idea to keep Bacitracin (a topical ointment used to prevent skin infections) in your BDSM disaster kit (in case skin does get broken). Some inventive kinksters have suggested massaging the ointment onto the buttocks before the caning even begins. (Arnica cream and vitamin K also help with healing damaged skin.)

With canes, it's a good idea to pre-negotiate how many strokes the sub will take *and* to give him or her breathing room between each stroke since it takes a few seconds to absorb the shock of a cane. With canes be *extremely* careful about where and how you deliver each stroke. For the inexperienced caner, stick to the buttocks (far from the tailbone). Once you have some experience, you can move onto the upper thighs, the upper back (far from the spine), and even the soles of the feet, assuming you do it lightly.

> ### Never flog or crack a cane on the toes or tops of the feet.
>
> Feet have tiny fragile bones. This practice of foot flagellation is known as *bastinado*. I knew some subs who hated it, but (perhaps because my feet are so calloused) I liked it. These same subs often mocked me for my inability to withstand any form of nipple torture . . . to each his own!

So how do you cane someone without making a bloody mess? Firstly, practice, not on your partner, but on an inanimate object. One website suggested draping a towel over a chair and caning said chair. If, like me, you happen to have a mannequin you found on the sidewalk, use that! (But put some pants on it for padding so you don't break your cane.) Now make sure there is some distance between you and that inanimate object, enough that you can deliver a whack with the flick of a wrist. Accuracy is important, so in the beginning, keep your elbow at your side and as you improve, you can start to add a little elbow.

How to take a caning? Lying face down, standing up, or (the most traditional position) standing and bent over a chair. However you position your body, make sure your ass cheeks are an easy target *and* make sure you breathe deeply throughout. That goes for all of the activities herein this tome—taking a spanking, a caning, or a flogging. As a sub, you always want to breathe into your lower belly and keep your body relaxed. Canes offer a sensation unlike anything else and they also mark unlike anything else, so if you happen to be married and cheating with a BDSM play partner, avoid them altogether lest you want your hubby or wifey to question the tiger stripes across your ass.

Starting the flagellation chapter with caning was not unlike starting an Introductory to Science textbook with quantum physics, so let's move onto some other, easier to handle flogging devices.

Popular Flogging Devices

Riding Crops—Oh, how I love riding crops! They *look* sexy, they feel great, and they make a cool sound. Probably one of the most versatile tools of the trade, they can be used almost anywhere on the body.

I distinctly remember that during one of my first sessions, a gentleman ran one over my shirt and my magic wands immediately perked up. He then slipped the riding crop under my shirt. It was cool and soft and he smacked my breasts lightly with it before running it over my jeans, eventually thrusting it between my legs. When he finally got around to smacking my ass with it, a puddle had begun to form beneath me. Years later, when I met a new lover and noticed he had a crop hanging over his door, I knew we would hit it off.

When using a crop, as with everything else, start slowly. Caress your sub's body with it. Maybe even make him or her kiss the crop. Basically get your sub hot and bothered before getting into it, building to some decent thwacks. We won't go fully into "sub training" for this book since it's a beginner's manual, but there are certain positions that are deemed appropriate for "taking" the crop or any other instrument for that matter.

The first position, "kneeling," involves simply going down on one's knees. "Arch," on the other hand, demands that the sub both kneel and lean back toward the floor. The "submissive position" involves kneeling while simultaneously bending forward, ass in the air. Finally, one performs "display position" by standing up with your hands behind your head. You will find a variety of names for these positions, and there are no hard and fast rules dictating submissive positions or behavior. If you are a sub, just thrust that ass in the air to show that you are enthusiastic!

Paddles—Paddles is a sweeping category. Traditionally, paddles come in two varieties: wood and leather. But . . . I have seen everything under the sun—Ping-Pong paddles, hairbrushes, seemingly innocent kitchen utensils, things that looked like boat oars, and even a picket from a white picket fence. (When you've been a sub or a Dom, it's tough to ever see a hardware store or even an office supply store the same way again.)

Paddles feel a lot like a spanking, but they spare the spanker's hand. Careful with them because they, too, can leave bruises—and if it's a wooden hairbrush, it's gonna hurt like hell. My favorite paddle was named "Pam." It was obtained by Mr. Hall, who bought it from 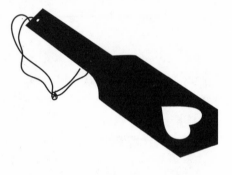 a sweet elderly woman at a yard sale. We believe a sorority used it in the '60s for "hazing" pledges.

Mr. Hall recounts, "I can't recall who I was fucking at the time, but we saw the paddle and HAD to have it. I tried to play normal by buying some pottery and then I asked about the paddle. Though in memory I thought it was for a fraternity, it seems that it's from a sorority. Anyway I purchased the paddle (and pottery) quite cheaply. Pam has several markings. On one side it says, 'Florida State' in large letters. In smaller letters are 'Gamma Phi Chapter, Jan. 25, '69,' something that appears to be a Florida State seal and the maker, 'Old hickory paddle co. DANVILLE IND.' The other side also has a seal, the Alpha Omega symbols, and the name, 'PAM.' I love Pam." Since then, Pam has seen a lot of action.

Slappers—A slapper is a lot like a paddle, only it consists of two pieces of leather, sewn together. It makes a sound much like slapping, hence the name.

Single-Tailed Whips—There are a few varieties of single-tailed whips, with the bullwhip being the most popular, or at least the most recognizable. Other types include blacksnakes, stock whips, buggy whips, and signal whips. These mothers are not easy to use. Keep in mind that the longer the whip is, the harder it is to control, thus increasing the risk of injury. The best way to learn to use a single-tailed whip is from someone who already *knows* how to use one. And believe it or not, the Internet is full of instructional videos on how to use a whip. (Less creepy than researching spanking online.)

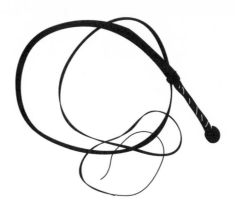

The "forward crack" is the simplest stroke to deliver. To perform this, hold the whip with your dominant hand and let the whip lay perfectly straight, trailing behind you. If you don't keep the whip straight, it could result in whipping your own leg. (Uncool!) Now swing your arm forward and up. Your hand should come up to your shoulder, with your palm facing your body and your elbow aimed at your target. Return downwards to your side. Continue swinging up and down, but don't crack it yet! During the upswing, the whip should fully and firmly extend, then create a loop to make a pop. If you follow the steps accurately, the whip makes a loop at the top of the upswing, right as you bring the whip out towards the target.

Again, solo practice is encouraged. One good rule of thumb when first learning to crack a whip is to keep your feet planted firmly on the ground and to move only your arms. Practice on stuffed animals or pillows, really anything that isn't a human, and when you finally try it with a partner, check for clearance! I just read a story online (while tirelessly researching this book) about a dude who went to whip his ladylove and got his bullwhip caught in the overhead ceiling fan. The fan subsequently fell on his sub. Luckily, no major injuries occurred.

Multi-Tailed Whips—Again, this is a diverse group of implements. All multi-tailed whips deliver something of a thud *and* a sting, but each varies depending on how it's made. The sting factor is decided mostly by the type of hide you are using, whereas the thud usually depends on how thick the hide is and how many tails it has. A general rule of thumb is that the fewer tails a whip has, the more it will sting, whereas a whip with a lot of tails can almost feel like a deep tissue massage.

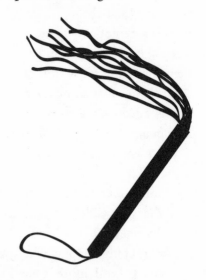

The general term for most multi-tailed whips is *flogger*. There are a million types of floggers, combining different tails and handles. The most popular amongst them is the cat o' nine tails (often just called "the cat.") It's about 76 cm long and comprised of nine knotted thongs of cord. It was originally designed to lacerate the skin and cause intense pain. Like everything else on this list of devices, it was historically used for punishment (mostly against slaves) until pervs found out how much fun it was. Its shorter cousin is the French "martinet," which is made of a wooden handle of about 25 cm in length and about 10 lashes of equal, relatively short length.

Using a multi-tailed whip is much easier than using a single-tail. (If I can wield one, chances are, you can, too!) A simple horizontal whack works well on the buttocks when one's partner is bent over and sticking them out while a vertical stroke works well on the shoulder blades. A "figure 8" move is also relatively easy to master, as is a propeller move wherein you spin the tails around in a circle from your wrist and then bring them up against your partner's booty. For more of a sting, flick the tails against your partner's buttocks as you would a wet towel in a locker room.

If you shop for floggers online, you will likely find that many of them are made of leather (and are pricey). If you are a vegan or just a poor person, don't panic! Just head (again) to Home Depot and pick up some rubber tubing or rope. It's quite easy to make your own. I even found someone online who made a flogger using two used bike inner tubes, scissors, a scalpel, ruler, and pen. (The scalpel wasn't entirely necessary.) I won't describe the exact process for making your own because this isn't an arts and crafts book, and because I don't want to bore you to tears, but just know that there are many vegan pervs out there who have shared detailed instructions online.

Straps—A *strap*, sometimes also called *strop*, is exactly what it fucking sounds like: a strap of something, usually leather. It's a lot like a paddle and should be used much like a paddle, though (unlike a paddle) it will likely have a little bend to it, so be careful it doesn't wrap around to a vulnerable body part.

Belts—Pilgrims once wore these on their hats, but now people worldwide have discovered that belts a) hold your pants up and b) can be used to erotically "torture" subs in BDSM play. Much like using a strap, be careful of them wrapping around your partner's body, especially because of their length. You don't want to aim for the ass and get the pudenda or lower abdomen.

As you can see, learning to flagellate someone properly is a little like training for a triathlon—no easy task. But the rewards (your sub's undying devotion and horniness) are well worth the effort.

Fetishes

Switching gears, let's talk about fetishes. If you were to have asked the mythical creatures known as Masters and Johnson how many fetishes exist on Earth, they would likely have responded "as many as there are stars in the sky." No one understands this better than me, who, as a sex columnist, risked carpal tunnel weekly, trolling the web searching for new fetishes to write about. It seemed no matter how many I discovered one day, there were always more the next.

As mentioned earlier, I once attended a "balloon fetish" party where I jumped inside a giant balloon. What I didn't mention is that the AirVac hose pumping air into the balloon became detached and I almost suffocated as the balloon started shrinking around me. Hence I can safely say I risked the most ridiculous death ever researching fetishes.

What exactly is a fetish?

Sexual fetishism, or erotic fetishism, is the sexual arousal a person receives from a physical object or from a specific situation. The object or situation of interest is called the *fetish*; the person who has a fetish for that object/situation is a *fetishist*.

Most commonly, fetishes simply enhance sex, as with the boot fetishist I dated. When he gave me black PVC thigh-high boots and I wore them while we made love, it most certainly increased his arousal. (And I got cool boots out of it!) But we could still have great sex even if I was wearing old socks with holes in them. Like most fetishists, he was still interested in regular ol' intercourse, but his fetish just spiced it up a bit.

Arousal from a particular body part is called *partialism*. While feet are overwhelming the most popular "part" amongst fetishists, the list is long—legs, butts, necks, ears, breasts, and armpits all do it for some folk.

Paraphilia is yet another term, which means sexual arousal to objects, situations, or individuals that are not part of normative stimulation. Currently, a paraphilia is not diagnosable as a psychiatric disorder unless it causes distress to the individual or harm to others.

Fetishes and BDSM

Fetishes have a big role in BDSM play. Anton LaVey (founder of the Church of Satan) once said, "Every man is a fetishist. You simply have to *discover* his fetish." If a person has a fetish, it's usually not too hard to discover what it is. If you think he or she may be into feet, tell him/her your feet are damn tired and could use a massage. A foot fetishist will jump at the opportunity.

There are also other clues. Because I am an A cup, I will likely not attract a man with a "huge breast" fetish. (Though there are people with "small breast" fetishes, too!) Because I live in a six-floor walk-up, and therefore have seriously toned stems along with a penchant for micro-minis, I attract leg fetishists like bees to honey.

Since this is not a book about *why* people have fetishes or are into BDSM, I'm just going to list a few along with some minor notes. To keep research on the topic fun, I consulted not only my personal experiences and several BDSM guidebooks, but also my three thousand Facebook friends—none of whom are sexologists, but all of whom are over-sharing freaks.

Perhaps you and your partner can take a look at this list and circle the ones that excite you. If you have a fetish that your partner doesn't share or vice versa, it's not the end of the world. Most fetishists are not so extreme and an unwillingness to indulge their fetish generally doesn't mean it's over. When given the choice between a partner and a fetish, the overwhelming majority of people would choose their partner. But fetishes can be fun, especially if cool outfits are involved. With that said, I present you with a fun-filled yet totally incomplete list of fetishes.

My Friends' Fetish List

High heels and knee-high boots

Leather, latex, and rubber

Ball stretching

Cages (being locked inside 'em!)

Piercings

Hair

Smoking

Hips

Flannel

Bunions

Schoolgirl uniforms (As a sub, this is basically *all* I wore.)

Bunny ears (on women)

Little Red Riding Hood costumes

Superheroes

Giants (*Macrophilia* is the technical term for men who get off on the thought of 50-foot women.)

Adult babies (technically known as *infantilism*)

Catsuits

Being auctioned off for charity

Gloves

Wrestling

Voyeurism

Tickling

Age-Play

Threesomes

Exhibitionism

Balloons (Balloon fetishists are called *looners.*)

Feet (and all the other aforementioned body parts)

Enemas (giving and/or getting them)

Pony play

Farts

Shit

Piss

Blood

Snot

Fucking stuffed animals (These people are known as *plushies.*)

Furverts (Unlike *furries* who just enjoy wearing animals costumes, *furverts* get off on it.)

Vorarephilia (Arousal occurs from the idea of eating, or being eaten by, another person, or by an animal. Since the fetish generally cannot be carried out in real life, it is enjoyed through pictures, stories, and videos.)

Realistic blow-up dolls and robots (Also called *agalmatophilia*, this one is costly!)

Sploshing (Also called wet and messy fetish or WAM, it is a form of fetishism whereby a person becomes aroused when substances are deliberately and generously applied to the naked skin.)

A "car and sign" fetish (My friend, George *swears* he met someone with this fetish. . . .)

Chains, Whips, and Cuffs

And . . . vampires? I imagine, given the success of *Twilight* and the hotness of Robert Pattinson and Kristen Stewart, this fetish scene has grown. But vampires are not always glamorous. My friend Kat and I once attended a vampire fetish party in Brooklyn hoping to find something akin to the Cullen family. What we found instead was a sprinkling of cape-clad dorks, discussing computer technology. "I had a feeling," Kat said. "In nerd evolution, vampirism comes right after Dungeons & Dragons."

Finally, from my friend Dan: "A woman in a PVC costume spanking a tied-up latex model of a large freshwater leech (about the size of a person, and visibly breathing) wearing a polyester girdle and a single and very large shiny spiked heel to fit over its posterior—with a bubble machine and the theme to Godzilla droning in the background to set the mood."

Did I mention I have some very odd friends?

When a fetish involves a costume or make-believe scenario, it generally leads to our next topic. . . .

Role-Play

The role-play I refer to here is not Dungeons & Dragons, LARP, or World of Warcraft, but rather *sexual role-play* wherein two or more people act out a scenario that they find sexually stimulating. Role-play can be a fun form of foreplay where partners can get lost in "roles" and shed some sexual inhibitions. After a hard day at the orifice (ha!), sometimes this escape from reality is needed. Role-play is not exclusive to BDSM, but it's an important component in that most often the roles acted out involve a power dynamic like nurse/patient or captive/torturer.

But let your imagination run wild, as role-play gives your creative spirit a chance to shine. In my personal life, I've enacted everything from mermaid/fisherman to The Great God Pan/woodland nymph and more. (It helps that I have a lot of costumes.) And that's just in my personal life.

Professionally, within the course of a few hours, I would play a student being paddled by the principal for smoking, a horny teacher seducing her delinquent pupil, and an aspiring gymnast fending off her pervy coach. There were days when I adopted so many personalities, I felt like Sybil.

If you're new to role-play, nervous about it, and don't happen to have crates of costumes at your disposal, don't worry. Role-play is not about winning an Emmy or studying the Meisner Technique; it's about letting go. If you aren't sure where to begin, here are a few fave raves of role-play enthusiasts to get you started.

Common Roles to Play

Master/slave—This is the most basic form of BDSM role-play. A classic, it's like the Chanel No. 5 of kink. In it, the sub player is treated as the property of the Master or Mistress.

Age-Play—Here, one individual acts and/or treats another as if he or she is a different age. You could be a babysitter and your partner an unhappily married husband and father. (I said "unhappily" to make this less creepy.) *Infantilism* is an extreme form of age-play wherein one partner pretends to be a baby and the other a "mommy" or "daddy." They even make adult-sized cribs for those especially dedicated to this one.

Please note!

Role-play is simply a *game* in the magical, kinky world of make-believe that is BDSM.

If the fantasy involves some form of age-play a la principal/student and you are the Dom (playing the principal, I assume), it doesn't make you a sick fuck who will prey upon students in real life.

Alien/Abductee—I'll never forget my first day at the dungeon, when I entered the medical room and saw alien masks. *"What* are those for?" I asked Velocity. "Oh, those are for men who have alien abduction fantasies," she said nonchalantly. "Doms wear them when they torture them. They probably anally probe them and stuff."

Animal-Play—This is when one player is treated as an animal such as a dog, kitten, or pony. I actually got to "be" a kitten in one session and it was fun and liberating, meowing and rolling around on the ground. I imagine being a pony is harder since equestrian fetishists often ride around on their ponies. As is the case with having a *real* dog, being the Master of a sub who wants to be your dog is hard work (as we already covered in the "Can I Just Have a Sandwich?" section).

Torturer/Captive Prisoner—Here, one player is a captor who abuses the other. One need not look further than cult sexploitation movies of the '70s for inspiration here. *Ilsa, She Wolf of the SS* comes to mind. (Though many people find it disturbing and Ilsa castrates her captors for the crime of ejaculation in said film. Do not go that far! And no waterboarding!)

Kidnapping Fantasy—There are so many variations here! In this one, the submissive player is bound, possibly gagged, and teased. You could even add a "pirate twist" wherein the Dom is Bluebeard and the sub is the kidnapped wench. If you like Mafia movies, throw that in there. Perhaps your sub is a sultry informant and you got wise and are going to have your way with her. I once did a session where I was a witch and my "captor," an inquisition leader.

Gender-Play—Here, one or more players take on roles of the opposite sex. I make an extraordinarily ugly man and would be disturbed if anyone wanted anything to do with me whilst I am "Steve-A-Rino," my male alter ego. However, I get a kick out of putting makeup on men and dressing them up in wigs and gowns. (Straight men are rarely good at caring for wigs. *Never* lend them a wig they won't take care of or a dress that doesn't have a little stretch to it.)

In my experience, gender-play is one of the most commonplace desires submissive men harbor. Maybe because men's clothing is so boring. Plenty of Doms have told me stories about their subs simply wanting to dress in frilly lingerie. My friend "Mistress Victoria" had one sub (a corporate executive, of course!) who wanted to dance around her apartment while dressed in women's lingerie. As he was in the midst of dancing, he wanted her "manly boyfriend" to walk in and scream "What the hell is going on here?" so that he (the sub) could then cower in fear. At the time, Victoria was dating a well-known musician who was about 130 pounds and the opposite of macho. Still, he agreed to participate and threw on a pair of aviators and a "wifebeater" tank top. According to him, while not erotic, it was an extremely fun, albeit bizarre, experience wherein he could not keep a straight face.

Medical Fantasies—Much like the kidnapping fetish, there are a mind-boggling number of variations here. Old-fashioned nurse's getups, speculums, enemas (a load of information on them later!), and gynecological tables all fall under this umbrella term for a fetish involving doctors, nurses, and patients. Perhaps you are the English

Patient, totally infirm and bedridden, and a super hot Juliette Binoche-type nurse is caring for you (i.e., blowing you). Or maybe you are a submissive patient and your hot doctor or nurse is a torturer! Maybe he or she asks you to take off all your clothes for a "thorough" examination. (Personally I'd like to role-play having health insurance, but that's way off subject.)

Uniforms—Uniforms are hot for many reasons. They generally represent authority, discipline, dignity, and power. As many women have pointed out, they also mean the wearer has a job. And not to be sexist, there are plenty of men who find a woman in a uniform sexy. Seeing Beyoncé don a cop uniform for the "If I Were a Boy" video, I concur. As a friend recently said to me, "When I see a cop, all I think about is that billy club." When I asked this friend if security guards did it for him, he said, "That's for S&M light."

Uniform role-play can get costly depending on your getup of choice, but if you and your lover are savvy, you'll have fun rummaging through thrift stores looking for great finds that might inspire whatever is in store later that night. For a few bucks, one can be a cheerleader, an army guy, a cop, a football player, a nun (okay, maybe can't find that in a thrift store), a Sailor Moon girl, or any number of members of The Village People. As the sub, you can be the arrestee, a shoplifter, or really any sinner of your choosing.

Rape Play or "CAN"—This is where one player feigns being coerced into an unwelcome sex act. Sometimes it is referred to as "consensual non-consent." Mr. Hall came up with a new name for it—Consensually Arranged Non-Consent or CAN for short. This form of role-play is controversial and rarely written about, probably out of fear that real-life rapists will view it as a "see, she wanted it" excuse. But we are talking about *role-play* and *fantasy*.

> If the role-play scenario involves a rape fantasy, it does not mean that the Dom actually *wants* to rape someone or that the sub *wants* to be raped in real life. So don't hate yourselves for enacting whatever turns you on.

In fact, rape fantasies are not uncommon in women. For some women who were raised in households where sexuality was a taboo topic, being the sub in a rape fantasy gives them the freedom to be "ravished" and "corrupted" through no fault of their own. If you just now opened this book for the first time and happened to turn to this page, please go back and read the "Safety First" section and make certain, before engaging in CAN, that you and your partner understand the *consensual* part and that you have pre-negotiated and made arrangements ahead of time.

For example . . .

I cannot stress pre-planning enough when it comes to CAN. As Mr. Hall said, "The 'arranged' part is important for avoiding danger and getting your scene to sing. That is, unless you want to wind up in the hospital after your partner punched you in the face because he or she didn't know it was you under that ski mask or wind up in jail because you thought public abduction in a tinted van would be hot. It is highly recommended that you arrange a time, place, and a few other details in advance of your CAN."

Mr. Hall went on to further describe a CAN experience he and his ladylove had where things didn't go as planned:

"My partner and I had discussed CAN many times. We shared our fantasies and our fears, established our boundaries, and had long ago chosen our safe words. Finally the time had come!

"We agreed that this would occur at her apartment when she arrived home from work that day. I was going to hide inside near the door, grab her and thrust her over the couch, then ravish her while lifting her skirt and tearing off her thong. I'd then hold her down and fuck her senseless as she struggled and protested.

"The first small impediment to our plan was the unplanned early arrival of her little red bastard (slang for 'menstruation'), so I placed a towel over the couch. Better to lose a touch of the fantasy than to ruin expensive furniture. She texted to let me know she was almost home and I wrote back, 'I had to run some errands and might have forgotten to lock the door ;)' She replied, 'I'm sure nothing bad will happen ;).' I was rock hard and ready to pounce when I heard the door start to open.

"Then I saw two large bags of groceries in her hands. Though she would have been fine with the bags, she hadn't taken into account how retentively clean I tend to be. There was no way I could risk a stained rug or even allow perishables to go un-refrigerated for however long our CAN session might have been.

"After I helped her put away the groceries, it was agreed that the moment was lost. We still fucked each other senseless, but the next time we chose to play CAN, we were a bit more detail-oriented and it was as hot as CAN can be (really, really super hot)!"

Hopefully, these tips have been helpful and Mr. Hall's story illustrates how important communication is. No matter how excited you are by your kink, you always put *being a human* first. This, means, among other things, being willing to drop whatever fantasy has you rock hard or soaking wet, for just a moment, to put all the groceries away.

Let's move onto less controversial role-play scenarios!

Stripper Fantasy—When working as a sex columnist for *Nerve*, I went "undercover" as a stripper at Wiggles, one of the only all-nude joints left in New York City. For the assignment, Velocity gave me a pair of 6-inch pink Lucite heels and a hot pink baby-doll negligee. These I wore, not only to Wiggles (where I had a very bad attitude as a stripper), but also into the bedroom where I gave my boyfriend at the time a lap dance. Sadly, he put no bills in my thong. In fact, he was kind of a jobless scumbag who was eating me out of house and home at the time (and not in a good way). But we did have many nights of great sex and that evening was particularly steamy. (By many nights, I mean four years. I have since realized there are decent, employed men who eat you out, but leave you with the house and home.)

Librarian Fantasy—Who hasn't fantasized about a sexy librarian or even a "manbrarian" for that matter? How 'bout one partner be the sub who has a bunch of overdue library books or worse—tries to steal a library book—and one partner be the dominant librarian who delivers punishment for such horrid transgressions? The Dewey Decimal System's never been hotter! (Side note: I have actually dated a "manbrarian" and he had a huge package and excellent oral skills. He also obtained a copy of Cher's *The First Time* for me. Never overlook the shy types!)

Owner/Inanimate object—Once again, I'll bring up the "Can I Just Have a Sandwich?" type of relationship. Though this fantasy does not have to entail the 24/7 lifestyle, it does, for the sub, involve being an "owned inanimate object," such as a desk your Dom might write a letter on. If you are hyperactive like me, being human furniture or even sitting still for a few minutes (unless I'm tied up) is nearly impossible. In fact, this might be the least active form of role-play there is.

The "correct" term for human furniture (a person getting off on pretending to be furniture and someone else getting off) is *forniphilia*. I have found examples in art, in magazines, and online of men and women "being" table lamps, coffee tables, bookshelves, hat and key racks, and more. The web site House of Gord (www.houseofgord.com) offers supreme examples of this, ranging from a "human rooster weather vane" atop a barn to a "human garden swing."

Because forniphilia is an extreme form of bondage wherein one partner is usually bound and expected to stay immobile for a prolonged period, frequent checks of the submissive should be done to make sure your beloved table, chair, or hat rack is A-OK. Since we're on the subject of forniphilia, a *forniphilic gag* is a type of gag that has the primary purpose of objectifying and/or humiliating the wearer. It is usually a mounting point for a tool or other device, which allows subs to perform tasks or services for their Doms. When using the gag, the slave's hands are usually bound behind the sub so he or she has no other option than to control the tool with the gag, be the tool a toilet brush, ashtray, dildo, or vibrator.

Chains, Whips, and Cuffs

Prison Fetish—As someone whose loving boyfriend just gave her a 3-DVD box set of Linda Blair "Women in Prison" movies, I can attest to the hotness of this role-play scenario. (Prison films are one of my favorite genres of cheese so I am something of an expert here.) While it might seem "prison fantasies" could only be something enacted between same-sex couples, I have discovered via *Chained Heat, Barbed Wire Dolls, Reform School Girls, Hellhole Women,* and more that there are many options. You could be seduced, degraded, or taken against your will (thus incorporating CAN) by a wicked guard, or you could reverse those roles and play a cunning prisoner who seduces the guard so that he/she will help you escape. *Or* you could play the court-appointed evil psychiatrist who seduces a prisoner. Or *maybe* enact an episode of *Scared Straight* where one of you is a juvie who gets "straightened out" by a hardened prisoner (thus working in age-play). The possibilities are limitless!

Client/Escort—Have you ever heard the saying "Men pay prostitutes to leave?" I've never really bought that one. I think men pay prostitutes to *be prostitutes*, to be the opposite of what "good girls" are. And as a woman who kind of looks like the girl next door (or the rapidly aging sleep-deprived forty-year-old next door), I know firsthand how sexy switching gears from "Mary Ann" to "Ginger" or "Sandy at the beginning of *Grease*" to "Sandy at the end of *Grease*" can feel. It's liberating to be a whore! (I should know.)

This is a fun scenario to act out at a cheap hotel if given the chance. If not acted out at a hotel, the partner who is the "escort" should get ready elsewhere and "arrive" at the location for authenticity's sake, even if it means getting ready in the house's bathroom, going out the backdoor, and then ringing the doorbell at the front door.

Of course, you first have to decide *who* is going to be the escort. Maybe he's an American Gigolo. Maybe she is a streetwalker. Maybe she's high-end. Maybe you are a same-sex couple and one of you is a powerful politician whose life would ostensibly be ruined if anyone were to find out. Either way, figure out a detailed scenario and an escort name. (Mine is "Trinity.")

Dress-up and dirty talk are both a big part of this one, so get gussied up and let your filthy mouth reign free. "Negotiate" what the client wants and what it'll cost him or her. Embrace the role even if it's awkward at first. You are taking on the world's two oldest professions—prostitution and acting!

Other Roles You May Want to Play. . .

Gangster/Someone paying off a gambling debt

Landlord/Slutty tenant who is facing eviction

Survivors of a zombie apocalypse

Survivors of a shipwreck

Repairman/Horny housewife

Hitchhiker/Driver

Robot/Master

Sleeping Beauty/Prince Charming

Model/Photographer

Goddess/Worshipper

Scientist/Horny Bride of Frankenstein

Santa/Naughty elf

Wizard/Elf

MILF/Young next-door neighbor

Cowboy/Cowgirl *or* Cowboy/Cowboy *or* Cowgirl/Cowgirl

Dastardly Whiplash/Ingénue tied to railroad tracks (obviously don't do this on real railroad tracks . . .)

These are some of the more popular scenarios. Researching the topic online, I found many creative people had suggested a whole lot more. A few are listed in this column.

As with so many activities mentioned in this book, the only limits are your imagination, you and your partner's boundaries, and legality.

Chains, Whips, and Cuffs

(As in . . . something involving public nudity might *seem* fun, but could land you both in jail—not fun!)

And let's not rule out three-ways. A good three-way only increases the amount of role-play scenarios one can enjoy since you have more "actors." Horny married couple/nymphet, queen and her servants, two cheerleaders and a quarterback, and so on. But beware with three-ways: Everyone has got to be on the same page. Most three-ways I've engaged in have been wonderful, but a few have ended in tears and disappointment because one party felt like a third wheel. In a three-way, everyone needs equal attention, and if the three-way happens to involve intercourse and your boyfriend or husband, make damn sure that when he comes, it's while he's fucking you. Condoms generally don't break when used properly, but the last thing you want is to watch a condom break while your boyfriend is fucking the waitress you both picked up at In-N-Out Burger. (Not that I speak from experience or anything. . . .)

Suffice to say, role-play is fun when played properly. Planning is key, and so is a willingness on behalf of both partners to go at it with total sincerity. It's a great way to "let go" and drop the tedium that reality too often provides.

Temperature Play

Thus far we've covered role-play, fetishes, flagellation, spanking, humiliation, dirty talk, and more . . . and that's just the tip of the iceberg. (Pun intended because we're about to talk about temperature play!)

Temperature play is an umbrella term for a bunch of BDSM activities that range from ice play to hot wax to fire play and even a little sado-botany with stinging nettles, hence this will be the longest chapter herein. We'll only briefly mention fire play toward the end of the book; this is where I'll discuss different forms of "edge play" (i.e., risky BDSM behaviors that this author wouldn't recommend—especially if you don't have health insurance or years of training as an EMT or doctor). However, there are some forms of temperature play that are a great way to "break the ice" when new to BDSM.

Ice (*It's hawt!*)

Ice does many things. It keeps our cocktails cold and, until it's entirely melted in the Arctic, it preserves our ecosystem and prevents the apocalypse thus furthering the expansion of the BDSM scene. Until that sad day when all the world's ice melts, we should try to appreciate it as much as we can (both the world and ice).

I first came to carnally appreciate ice accidentally. It was approximately 1991, well over 90 degrees, and my very first real lover and I had just destroyed my box fan during a spastic moment of overheated

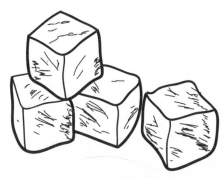

eroticism. Because I had no air conditioner, I ran to the freezer (where I frequently stuck my head at the time) and grabbed a cup full of ice, which I brought into the boudoir. Having never seen *Nine and ½ Weeks*, I had no real erotic intentions or idea of what to do with the ice, but pretty soon my lover and I were rubbing ice cubes all over each other. It started to melt quickly, as you could have fried eggs on both of our asses, and when I noticed he was popping wood, a little light bulb went off in my perverted head. Being inventive, I took an ice cube and inserted it into my vajayjay. Then my lover began to fuck me. The hot/cold/hot/cold effect made him crazy. That whole summer, ice cubes became a big part of our "too broke for air conditioning" fun. Some people go to cold movie theaters when they don't have AC, but I can't begin to recommend this enough. Just make sure the ice isn't filthy. Urinary tract infections and bacterial vaginosis are never fun. (Of course, anytime you put anything in your vag, you run the risk of infection, so make sure whatever goes in there is clean as an Irish spring.)

Painful, cumbersome vaginal infections aside, what else can you do with ice? If you are Zan, the Wonder Twin, you can transform into it! We are not all so lucky, but there is so much more. . . .

Stuff to Do with Ice that Doesn't Involve Cocktails

1. Ladies—Have your fella or your girlfriend place a cube in their mouth and go down on you.
2. Use ice post-sex during a massage, slowly running it up and down your partner's back.
3. Rub a cube between your teats and then guide your partner's member up and down the "cleavage slip and slide" you have created.
4. Just rub 'em up and down all over each other's bodies, as described earlier.
5. If one partner is blindfolded, you can alternate between pouring hot wax and trailing ice over his or her skin. (This is kind of an "advanced" exercise and should only be attempted with a familiar partner.) To get the same effect without a candle, you could heat up a towel and alternate caresses given between the hot towel and an ice cube.

---

6. Kiss each other while you exchange the ice cube. Play around with it, outlining each other's lips and face with it. As the ice cube gets smaller, search for it in your partner's mouth with your tongue.
7. Place a cube in your mouth as you run your tongue up and down your partner's manhood. (Not for the faint of heart or for cold winter nights where your landlord has turned off the heat.)
8. Reenact the scene from *Showgirls* where scummy director "Tony" humiliates Nomi by asking her to put ice on her nipples to make them hard.

For example . . .

Once again, I will hearken back to the days of yore when I was doing sessions with Annie. We had a particularly inventive client who liked to invent "games."

He handed Annie and I two heavy, hardcover encyclopedia-size books down from the bookshelf. He then instructed us to balance the books on our heads with our hands at our sides. Whoever dropped the book first would be the recipient of torture. Annie and I placed the books on our heads and tried to stand perfectly still, as he twisted our nipples and spanked our bottoms. Finally, Annie flinched, and her book came tumbling down. I beamed with joy since Annie had won every challenge in our last session with this client.

The client then told me to get a cup of ice from the kitchen.

"What should we do with the ice?" he asked me.

"We should put it inside of her."

Annie looked horrified, but in my delusional mind, I thought she might enjoy it, remembering the hot/cold/hot/cold fucking I'd had with my first boyfriend. However, that ice play had been in the summer, and this was mid-March. While we were in a heated room, the very idea of ice coming into contact with her pussy made Annie cringe.

But a deal's a deal, and after I'd fetched a cup of ice, Annie took an ice cube, put it inside a condom and slowly began to insert it. By the time it disappeared inside her, she was covered in beads of sweat.

Not long after, Annie exacted her revenge. The client told us to stand up and face each other. When we did, he produced two large nipple clamps and affixed them to our right nipples. He then somehow produced a piece of yellow string, which he used to attach the nipple clamps to each other. On the ground between Annie and me, he placed a paper towel.

"We're going to have a tug-of-war!" he announced. "Whoever crosses this line will lose," he added, pointing to the paper towel.

This was going to be my comeuppance for the ice scenario since I loathe nipple torture and Annie clearly loved it. Plus, her breasts were twice the size of mine. As she began to pull, I feared my entire mammary gland would become detached from my body. I mouthed the word "bitch" to Annie, who smiled.

Finally, I said, "I surrender before I lose what little breasts I have." Stepping over the paper towel, I accepted defeat. It was like a perverse episode of *Survivor.*

The client then told me to lie down on the leather bed. I did as instructed and he cuffed my wrists and ankles to the bed so I couldn't move. Meanwhile, Annie blindfolded me so I wouldn't know what was coming next. From this point on, I couldn't tell which hands were performing which act, the exception being when Annie stroked my hair and I recognized her gentle touch.

Nipple clamps were soon attached to my already sore nipples. I then felt a device called a Wartenberg Wheel trailing across my belly. The Wartenberg Wheel was originally designed by Dr. Robert Wartenberg to test nerve reactions, as it is rolled systematically across the skin. It has since been adopted by the BDSM community as a wacky toy used for sexual hijinks. The small wheel, which sits at the end of a short, usually stainless steel handle, features sharp, radiating pins that rotate around when rolled across the flesh.

While not sharp enough to pierce the skin unless excessive force is used, they occasionally hurt like a motherfucker, especially when you're tied up and wearing heavy nipple clamps.

(Now onto the ice part . . .)

But that was just the beginning. In case you're wondering what happened to the rest of the ice I'd procured, pretty soon a large ice cube, a mini-glacier of sorts, was thrust inside my pussy.

Is it possible to get frostbite on one's vagina? I panicked.

One set of hands then dumped the rest of the ice on my skin and trailed the various cubes up and down my body while the other set of hands lit a candle. I know because I heard matches being lit and smelled the scent of sulfur and dripping candle wax. Seconds later, a torrent of *hot* wax poured onto my *freezing* skin.

The prickling wheel, the ice, the wax, and the nipple clamps sent me into a transcendental state wherein my etheric body said "fuck this" and began to climb out of my physical body. But then, a vibrator set at full speed was thrust against my clit, and I was forced out of my momentary transcendence, not by sexual arousal, but by a neurotic fear of electrocution, given the close proximity of the ice to the electrical vibrator.

Just as I became convinced that I was about to die one of the lamest deaths in history, the vibrator did the trick and I had a fan-fuckin-tastic orgasm.

Hot & Cold

When a sub is tied or blindfolded and in that transcendent sub-space, he or she often won't be able to tell the difference between hot and cold, so the use of hot wax (to be covered next) and ice together can make for a phenomenally erotic experience.

I've also heard of people using melted butter (careful it's not too hot), melted chocolate syrup (again, careful), and refrigerated whipped cream during sex and BDSM. Who can forget the famous scene in *Last Tango in Paris* where Brando uses butter as anal lube? Though, having looked into this, butter as lube is *not* the best idea. Do yourself a favor and get some real lube.

My favorite is Pjur, a German lubricant. On the bottle it says, *"Klebt garantiert nicht,"* which is now the only German phrase I know. It means, "guaranteed never sticky." But because *Pjur* is pricey, I often opt for Liquid Silk. While a lot of folk like flavored lube, I shy away from it after a five-pack of Wet flavored lube exploded on my bed and my comforter smelled like grape flavored Kool-Aid for a month.

Also, if you do use any butter, olive oil, massage oil, or chocolate during BDSM play, keep it out of the vag or urethra. As I've said before, a UTI is no walk in the park. Actually with a UTI, you *can't* walk in the park because you will have to pee every five seconds.

Some BDSM enthusiasts also enjoy playing with pain relief creams such as Icy Hot, BenGay, and Tiger Balm. As Velocity gave me my first tour of the dungeon, I noticed a jar of Icy Hot sitting amongst the whips and chains. "What's Icy Hot doing here?" I asked.

"Some guys like to rub it on their balls. Whatever you do, don't ever let them rub it on your pussy."

Sound advice.

Yet another way to have fun with temperature play is through the use of glass dildos, which you can heat up or cool down. I first experienced a glass dildo during the Sex Toy Olympics, an event I created along with my friend Erin while I was working as a sex columnist. Erin had gotten a job as a sex toy reviewer and she'd been given so many toys, she had to outsource them to me. Many of these toys were glass dildos. Erin put the prettiest glass dildo, which featured a kaleidoscopic image of a flower, in the freezer.

"Don't forget it's in there," I warned her. "I don't think my roommate wants to discover that when he reaches for frozen tamales." When we finally pulled the dildo out of the freezer and popped it in my biscuit, it was too cold, causing the tongue-to-frozen-flag pole effect. That's when I learned you should cool your glass dildo with cold or ice water instead of placing it in the freezer.

Conversely, you should warm your glass dildo with warm or hot water right out of the tap for a few minutes. Using hot water ensures that the piece is equally warmed whereas microwaving your faux phallus can cause hot spots that can burn. If you've ever nuked a Mama Celeste pizza and bitten into it too soon, you know what I'm talking about. And there is absolutely no way you want that pizza-burn-on-the-roof-of-your-mouth sensation replicated within your vag or anus.

Wax Play (*Fun with Chemical Compounds!*)

Moving on, let's talk about wax! Like ice, wax serves many purposes. From crayons to creepy lifelike figures of celebrities, it's versatile. It is especially popular in BDSM, where its usage is referred to as wax play. This involves dripping hot wax from candles or ladling it onto a person's naked skin. It can be part of BDSM or just a part of plain ol' kinky sex. When done properly, it feels intense and erotic.

For example . . .

During my first session at the dungeon, "Pete" the "sword swallower" introduced me to hot wax as a kink.

"Have you ever had hot wax?" he whispered.

"No," I said, revealing my newness to the profession.

He scurried off and returned with a set of mammoth nipple clamps, which he clamped onto my tiny breasts. The clamps hurt, but I breathed deeply, trying not to fidget.

I stared into the mirrored ceiling and began to study myself. I still had tan lines and the thong was pushed down so low my pubic hair was almost visible.

"Close your eyes," he said.

While pretending to close my eyes, I glimpsed Pete lighting a candle. I wondered if he was going to remove the clamps before he gave me the hot wax.

He returned with a lit candle.

"Have you ever been spit on?" he asked.

"No."

Leaning in close, he spit, aiming for my breasts.

A globule landed on my clamp-clad right nipple. He spit again, aiming for the left. He rubbed the spit into my chest, which made the skin feel tight. (Spitting is yet another part of BDSM that likely falls under the "physical humiliation" category. It's not complex enough to earn its own section.)

In the mirror, I watched Pete lift the candle and tip it toward my breasts. He poured the hot wax over them and I screamed, more from shock than pain. He began drizzling hot wax over my entire body, finally bringing the candle near my face.

"Please, not my face," I begged, not wanting my eyeballs seared.

Turns out that I was right to be afraid. One of the number one rules of wax play is "not near the face or eyes."

With wax, there are other codes of conduct and different levels of play to be considered. Wax should feel intense, but it should also feel good. You should not feel like you have to call 911 afterward. Once I realized that Pete wasn't going to drip hot wax into my eyes, I settled in for the ride and relaxed into the tantalizing sensation.

Later I also found that picking and peeling dried hot wax off of my skin was fun, sort of like when you put glue on your hand as a child and then peel it off.

Be Safe!

When dealing with a burning hot substance, safety is extremely important. Luckily, by learning a few simple techniques and procedures, you can have lots of fun with wax without sending your loved one to the burn unit.

First, wax, while easy to peel off skin, is a huge pain in the ass to get out of clothing, sheets, or any kind of fabric, so before you begin make sure the wax recipient isn't wearing couture while reclining upon a sixteenth-century Persian silk carpet. Nudity or a "blank canvas" is preferred.

While fetish garments look hot, plenty will melt and stick to the skin, causing burns. Anything with nylon, vinyl, PVC, or other synthetic fabrics should be avoided. Have the waxee lie upon a tarp or some other disposable surface so you don't trash the place. Wax is *not* easy to get off of skin if that skin is extremely hairy. This is hardly an issue given the entire world seems to be either manscaping or womanscaping. But if you happen to be with a rare haired human, either avoid his or her hairy parts or rub a small amount of mineral/baby oil or lotion that contains *no alcohol* on the the body for easy wax removal. You can actually do this over your partner's entire body, massaging it in as part of the play. In fact, giving your partner a massage either before or after any physically intimate activity is a nice way to kick things off or wind your partner down.

Take a Hint from Tantric Sex

You will notice that I mention Tantric Sex throughout this book, not just because I'm a big fan of it, but because I also believe many of the precepts taught in Tantra can be applied to everyday relations with your lover. Things taught in Tantric Sex like giving your partner a massage before getting busy, looking in your partner's eyes, and taking your time are all things that can be applied to BDSM. These basic actions will make things that much hotter. Far too many people avoid eye contact while fucking, which is ridiculous. You aren't riding the subway at rush hour; you are fucking! So if you have your partner's penis in your mouth or perhaps your throat, take a minute to look up from your endeavor and into his eyes. And the same goes for if you are dining on her pink meat sandwich. Look up! Eye contact is hot.

Getting back to hair, if you have long hair on your head, pull it back in a ponytail. If wax does get in your hair, use a flea comb and some conditioner to get it out. Also, keep in mind that if you are the waxer, wax splashes, so careful with your getup too. You don't have to wear a hazmat suit, but maybe avoid wearing you favorite little black dress. Also, avoid any flowing clothing since flames will be involved. No bell sleeves!

How the waxee lies is up to both of you. Generally, I have reclined on my back when taking wax and it is dripped down my chest and stomach. I've also taken it while lying on my side where the wax sensually runs down the back and onto the breasts and stomach. You can also take it while lying on your stomach, so you can receive the dose of wax on the back and buttocks.

Now, don't just go to the 99-cent store and buy any crap candle. I'm not going to break down the exact temperature at which every type of candle melts, but there are some general guidelines when purchasing candles for wax play. Plenty of sex shops (where you can shop online with privacy) now sell candles made specifically for the purpose of wax play. The aforementioned Babeland (www.babeland.com) sells several that actually turn into massage oil, which softens the skin. Some specialty candles even come with a brush, which you can use to "paint" the wax onto the skin. Not to get too scientific here, but ideally, wax play candles should have the lowest melting point available, which is 125 to 135 degrees. However, plain white paraffin candles or household "emergency candles" are usually a safe bet, and the softer a candle is, the better—generally speaking. The inexpensive glass-jar pillar candles found in bodegas and botánicas have never failed me and they come in a brilliant array of colors.

Stay away from beeswax, oil-based candles, and gel jar candles because they burn the hottest. If you are using a soy candle, make sure your partner doesn't have a soy allergy. It's also not a bad idea to check for allergies before the fun begins by applying a small amount of wax to a small patch of skin. If there is any redness or irritation, use that candle for home décor, but not for play, as your partner could have an allergic reaction to whatever dye, perfume, or additives are in it. I also recommend using the candle on yourself before using it on another so you know how it feels, as you should with a flogger or any new BDSM implement.

When engaging in wax play, keep open flames away from the body and lit candles or a Crock-Pot (should you be melting a boatload of wax) on a stable, level surface. If you have cats, keep the little fuckers in a separate room so they don't go knocking the candles over. Also, keeping a damp cloth or towel and a fire extinguisher nearby in case of emergency is recommended.

Wax On

There are several ways to apply wax. I like the good old-fashioned dripping method. When dripping, hold the source of wax at least 18 inches above the skin to give the drips some time to cool. It's best to hold the candle horizontally rather than vertically. If you hold the candle vertically, it will drip too fast and not have time to cool before landing. Again, avoid the face, and be especially careful with delicate areas like the nipples, navel, and genitals.

So Lifelike!

Speaking of the genitals, I actually had my vulva cast in wax by a mad eccentric artist named Mangina who makes molds of vulvas, then casts the "negative" to make a replica of said vulva, which he wears onstage.

This complex process involved lying on an inclined surface (legs elevated) while Mangina "fluffed" me so that my mold would feature an impressive clit boner. He then cut open an aloe plant and rubbed the aloe juice on my vulva to avoid genital searing before pouring a large amount of hot wax onto my nether region. The result? A mold that led to wearable art!

Note: Mangina is an accomplished sculptor who's been making manginas for years. Don't try this at home. Though they do sell "Clone-A-Pussy" and "Clone-A-Willy" kits, they just aren't the same. In fact, I was recently given a "Clone-A-Pussy" kit, which my boyfriend filmed me using. The result was a disaster movie more epic than *The Poseidon Adventure*.

Getting back to wax application, aside from dripping, there are three other basic methods: pouring, painting, and layering. These three get complicated because they often involve the use of a Crock-Pot and, personally, I find anything involving kitchen equipment daunting. Luckily, one nice lady from Erotic Sensations, an online store that has a huge selection of wickless jar candles, posted video instructions online. These folks seem to be the real experts here and you can find inexpensive candles designed for wax play at their site, http://eroticsensations.us.

In said video, this "Julia Child of wax play" takes the lids off a bunch of colorful jars of paraffin wickless candles and carefully places them in a Crock-Pot, which she then pours water in *just up to the wax line*. She then turns it on high and, like most cooking shows, we jump ahead two hours. After two hours, the candles have all melted. To test the temperature she takes a little sponge on a stick and dips it in one of the candles, then rubs some of the wax on her arm. "Perfect!" she exclaims. The little sponge tool, she notes, is great for applying wax. "You could even write your name with it," she boasts.

The online instructor then shows how you can also scoop out the wax with a spoon or ladle and pour it on. Heat-resistant squirt bottles can also be used for a Jackson Pollock effect. Just don't squirt near the eyes!

In terms of "painting," you can use any type of non-metal bristle brush, but before using it, make sure the bristles do not melt in the wax and do not use wax that is higher than 125 degrees, since you'll be getting awfully close to the skin.

"Layering" is basically when you combine the previous methods and either pour, drip, or paint several layers on your partner's skin. This looks pretty, but be warned—that much wax can retain heat, so frequently check in with your partner while you create your masterpiece to make sure he or she is safe.

Now wax on, wax off and keep that flame of lust burning.

Sado-Botany

I'm going to be perfectly honest here. I didn't even know a thing called sado-botany existed until I started researching this book. I'm including it in this section because if you've ever been rubbed with stinging nettles, you know that shit burns.

Stinging Nettles

The first time I endured this form of temperature play was in Bath, England, where I was attending a wedding with a lover who had a wonderful kinky side. As he and I walked around the lush, green grounds of the farm where the wedding was taking place, he pointed out the various types of butterflies and plants we passed. It was like being on a date with Richard Attenborough.

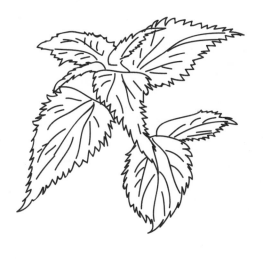

"Do you know what stinging nettles are?" he asked, plucking a plant from the ground.

"No."

"If you rub them on your skin, they sting," he said. "Here, hold out your arm. This is very cruel. People would probably get angry if they knew I were going to do this."

I held out my arm. (Thank God he never asked me to try heroin; I probably would've done it.) He rubbed the stinging nettle onto my arm.

"Oh man, it really stings. How long does it sting for?" I asked. It actually felt very much like hot wax.

"A while. We just need to find some dock leaves. There's one. It's been eaten away by caterpillars."

He plucked the dock leaf and rubbed it on my arm. Immediately the stinging stopped.

"When I was a kid, we used to chase each other with stinging nettles," he added.

After my experience in Bath, I tried to do a little research on stinging nettles, but all I could find was an episode of Dr. Oz where he said they could help treat seasonal allergies. I had no idea people were getting off on them. Yet, while researching temperature play, there it was: people actively using nettles as an instrument of erotic torment.

According to my research, nettles are best used in a gentle stroking or dabbing action, which will cause the "hairs" of the nettle (the tiny needle-like things on them) that come into contact with the recipient's skin to do the "stinging." Nettles are light enough to use for flogging, but be sure to check for allergies, as plant matter can be unpredictable. Most bodily areas are suitable for nettle play, but keep away from the face, of course, and careful with the penis, vaginal area, and anus.

Just when I thought I'd learned all there was to know about sado-botany, I uncovered more!

Figging

Even Mr. Hall was not aware of "figging" when I asked him about it.

"Does it have something to do with role-playing as Adam and Eve?" he asked.

Far from it, *figging* is the practice of inserting a piece of ginger root into the anus, vagina, or male urethra to cause an intense burning sensation. Originally applied to horses in a practice known as *gingering* (to make them "lively"), it now commonly refers to the aforementioned BDSM practice.

While ginger, when taken orally via healthy smoothies or tea, is good for you, figging has some risks. As is the case with sticking anything other than a penis up your ass, there is the danger of the ginger root entering the rectum completely and becoming irretrievable. That's why people who "fig" will often carve the ginger root into a butt-plug shape with a flared base.

A Good Rule of Thumb:

Anything you put in your ass should have a flared base.

Another Rule of Thumb:

Never put anything in your pussy that's just been in your ass. But we'll get to ass play later . . .

During my research, I also uncovered plenty of porn devoted to hot sauce being poured on women's pussies, often while they were tied up. The looks on their faces communicated to me that this is not pleasant, though I have never tried it. And I shan't judge lest I be judged.

There is a great likelihood that someone once fingered me shortly after he'd eaten nuclear wings and failed to use the Wet-Nap™ that accompanied them, but there are some things we choose to forget . . .

I will say that if you do get the wild hair up your ass to douse your pussy with hot sauce, as with all food products and oils, please *only* use it externally.

Sensation Play

Sensation play, like temperature play, is an umbrella term that describes activities meant to impart physical sensations upon a partner, as opposed to mental forms of erotic play such as role-play and humiliation. We've already covered some activities that are considered sensation play, like paddling and spanking, but there is so much more. Here we'll quickly go over a variety of activities and the instruments they entail. It should be noted that sensation play is often combined with bondage so that the sub is forced to surrender to the sensory experience at hand. *Also,* sensation play can involve heightening sensations *or* removing sensations. Usually it involves both at once, but we are going to start with sensory deprivation, namely blindfolds.

Instruments Used in Sensation Play

Blindfolds—It might seem hypocritical that only a few chapters ago, I encouraged readers to look into their partners' eyes and I 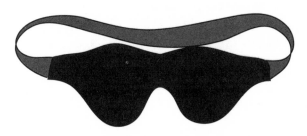 am now going to espouse the benefits of blindfolds. First of all, if you live in a crap apartment with east-facing bedroom windows, as I do, you know their value as sleep masks. In fact, I cannot sleep past dawn unless I have my blue satin "10 More Minutes Please . . ." sleep mask affixed to my head. But sexually speaking, blindfolds are hot. They are also a great way to ease into BDSM since they are generally inexpensive and unlikely to cause injury (assuming you aren't with a psycho).

Since blindfolds deprive you of sight, they enhance the remaining senses of the wearer, focusing attention on sound, smells, and physical contact. Anticipation of "what is coming next" is heightened, and I think we can all agree that one of the greatest things about sex is the *anticipation* of it.

Be sure to get a blindfold that fits. Because I have a pinhead, I've found that most blindfolds are too big for me and have used this to my advantage by cheating during piñata demolitions throughout the years. But when using one for kinky purposes, I want it to work.

For example . . .

During many professional sessions where I had access to fancy blindfolds, I would spend the entire hour in complete darkness. As mentioned previously, I was often blindfolded by Annie and led around on a leash to my Master. I was then asked to caress and undress him. Usually, while this occurred, both Annie and my Master would caress me, and I was unable to differentiate between male and female hands.

During one session, my Master, "Jeremy," had brought me a blindfold and a leopard print cat suit to wear. Once I put on the cat suit, Annie slipped the blindfold over my eyes and tugged on my leash, leading me to a suspension bar where she attached my wrists and raised the bar. She then tied my ankles to two posts on either side of me.

Jeremy flogged my upper back, alternating between a cat-of-nine tails and a horsetail whip. Meanwhile, Annie worked her fingers over my crotch, and I realized that Jeremy had strategically cut holes in the catsuit. She slipped a finger through a tiny hole in the crotch and played with my clit.

Jeremy ordered her to rip the fabric and she began to tear at it until my entire pussy was exposed. She worked two fingers inside of me, moving them in and out, while Jeremy dug his fingers into the fabric and tore the back open. I was completely disoriented (because of the blindfold), but it felt great.

He took Annie by her wrist-cuffs and attached her wrists to the bar, so that our bodies hung in suspension together. He continued to tear the fabric off me until my breasts were exposed. Annie's bra had been removed at some point and she thrust her pendulous breasts into my small, pointy ones. I bent my head down and licked them.

As you can imagine, I was eventually freed from suspension and moved to a leather bed where things got a little crazy (and technically illegal). My wrists were cuffed to posts over my head and my legs were tied in the air, spread eagle, to posts at either side of the bed. My two instructors mounted me and, I think, although my eyes were incapacitated, that the two gave each other oral sex over my inert body.

Annie's shaved pussy landed on my lips as she straddled my face.

"Lick my pussy," she said and I did as told.

Jeremy then chained Annie's wrists to a post over the bed so she was just a bit higher up than before, and I had to crane my head to satisfy her. She moaned, and I thought maybe she came. I was so caught up in what I was doing to Annie that I barely realized Jeremy doing his best to bring me to orgasm. His fingers were working on my g-spot and his tongue was on my clit.

Annie climbed off me, and all I could feel was a multitude of limbs and hands on my skin. Cold chains tickled me and fingernails dug into me. Gasps of pleasure filled the room. I heard someone unwrap a condom and in complete darkness I felt skin, tongues, stubble, hair, and teeth.

"Do you want to come?" Jeremy asked.

"Yes, Sir," I moaned.

"Do you want me to fuck you?"

"Yes, Sir."

"Say it."

"Please fuck me, Sir."

Jeremy entered me deftly, although with my legs tied spread eagle, I was an easy target. Annie played with my tits while he moved inside of me. Delirious, I reached climax before Jeremy, due to the fact that I had four hands, two tongues, and one penis stimulating me, and he only had one vagina—that's not to put down my vagina or to say that *he* had a vagina. It's just that my vagina had been over-stimulated to a point of no return. Though I'm not a screamer, it was so intense that I screamed. Jeremy continued pounding me until I came again.

If this quaint story doesn't say a lot for blindfolds, I don't know what will. Go out and get yourself one. If you have a nice silk scarf, you already have one!

No Blindfold At All—Sometimes, you don't need a blindfold at all. As the Dom, you can tell your sub to simply keep his or her eyes closed, as Mickey Rourke did to Kim Bassinger in *Nine and ½ Weeks*. During this fine scene, he feeds her what actually appears to be a revolting array of foods and substances including Vicks® couch syrup and gelatin (What? Were they in a hospital?) but at least she gets some champagne and strawberries before he coats her in honey and bangs her brains out.

Ear Plugs—Just as blindfolds are used to limit a sub's vision, ear plugs can be used to deprive a sub of his or her sense of hearing. They are not used that often because, presumably, subs want to hear what their Masters have to say.

Erotic Tickling—This one is kind of sweet. *Obviously* it involves people getting off on tickling or being tickled. Occasionally there are public tickling games or contests, which test the ticklee's endurance to being tickled, for amusement, for erotic pleasure, or for other reasons. Usually the recipient of the tickling is bound or blindfolded. I really enjoy this one but am too afraid of pissing myself to really get into it.

Gags—Like fetishes, there are as many types of gags as there are stars in the sky, but they all serve one very important purpose: They shut another person the fuck up for a brief moment in time.

Gags, like most other fetish toys, also increase the Dom's sense of power and the sub's sense of helplessness, hopefully heightening the intensity of the erotic escapade at hand. Some fetishists get off on the drooling along with the muffled sounds the sub makes while gagged, while still others get off on the visual aspect of the gag. In the case of the open-mouth gag, the accessibility of the wearer's mouth for doing what thou wilt may please the Dom.

Gags fall into three main categories: over-the-mouth, mouth stuffing, or mouth opening. On Wikipedia alone, twenty-three varieties of gags are listed, though there are certainly hundreds more. The most popular and enduring is the ball gag, which is usually made of 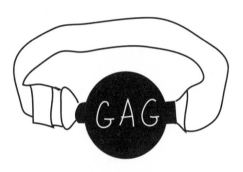 rubber or silicone in the shape of a sphere. There are penis-shaped gags so you can literally straddle and fuck your lover's face, and then there are inflatable penis gags so you can straddle and fuck your lover's face as the penis attached to their face inflates inside of you. Conversely, there are penis gags where the faux penis goes inside the gagged sub's mouth *and* there are double-penis gags where the sub's mouth is gagged with a small dildo while the Dom fucks the larger dildo on the outside. Just what will they come up with next?!

There are the aforementioned forniphilic gags, also called "humiliator gags" (that come with attachments for ashtrays and toilet brushes), "pony bit" gags, dental gags, ring gags, and several varieties of open-mouth gags that allow your sub to blow you.

Interestingly enough, Mr. Hall suggested that it's quite possible and economical to make your own gag. This "Martha Stewart of BDSM" bought a two-dollar conical dog toy then, using a leather hole puncher, punched two holes in each side of it. He then strung rope through the holes and voila—a gag!

As with everything else, be careful. Both gags and hoods, which block the mouth, can become asphyxial hazards if the subject vomits or the nose becomes blocked. Yet another reason not to go chugging Jäger before a session . . .

Hoods—Hoods scare a lot of people thanks to *Pulp Fiction*'s "the Gimp." But hoods are really nothing to be afraid of as long as they are worn with the sub's safety in mind. Velocity Chyaldd recently directed me to Extreme Restraints' website (www.extremerestraints.com) where I uncovered more hoods than I ever thought possible—total sensory deprivation hoods, animal-shaped hoods, gas mask hoods, less daunting lightweight hoods, and something called a "Cum Bucket Hood," which features a urinal-style front that you can fill with whatever you wish. Because this hood has an open-mouth, your partner will have to be subjected to whatever you fill in the trough.

Nipple Clamps and Toys—My nipples are more sensitive than the soul of the most existential, angst-ridden acoustic folk guitarist on the planet, hence I *really* cannot handle nipple clamps for extended wear. Because I am an eternally braless hippie, not a day goes by that my boobs don't announce "Turkey's done!" to anyone within eyeshot.

Weirdly, when I've been in love and my lover has busted out the clamps for use on me, I've enjoyed them. This is going to sound cheesy, but when you really fall for someone, it's easier to take more pain and truly get off on it. Why? Because you love them! Simple enough. But that's all I'm gonna say about love. This book is not about finding love, keeping love, or marrying a love. It's not *The Rules* but rather all about *breaking the rules*—being a bad girl or boy, getting kinky, and clamping things onto your tits or pectorals or the tits and pectorals of others.

As with the other "toys," there is a mind-boggling array out there and not all of them are "clamps." Some are gentler, such as battery-operated nipple vibrators and "nipple suckers," which are soft, pliable little suction cups you can place on your teats to make them more sensitive. In terms of clamps, my wonderful group of perv friends all agreed that broad tip adjustable nipple clamps (that have the little screws) are the best, offering just the right amount of pinch and not too much pain. You can always add little weights if it's just not enough. They also agreed "alligator clamps" are by far the most painful because they have "teeth" like tiny gators.

Of course, you don't have to go out and buy fancy-pants nipple clamps. I once had a client use metal binder clips from Staples on my boobs. A twelve-pack is only $3.99. Better yet, steal them from the office and stick it to The Man! Now let's move on to a similar device—clothespins. They have so many uses, they almost deserve their own goddamned chapter.

Clothespins—Clothespins are generally thought of as fasteners used to hang clothing from a clothesline, but gaffers, grips, electricians, and production assistants also use them to hang shit on film sets. But that's not all! Clothespins are also the poor man's answer to the nipple clamp.

As somebody who (as explained earlier) has a low tolerance for pain regarding nipple play, I can offer one bit of advice to subs who want to please their nipple- 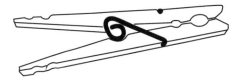 torture-happy partners: *Wooden* clothespins hurt a hell of a lot more than plastic ones. Not sure what mechanics are behind this, but it's true. I would rather ten plastic clothespins on my teats than one wooden one.

Moving along, clothespins aren't just for nipples. They can be placed pretty much anywhere you find loose flesh. One of the most painful sensations I've ever experienced was a wooden clothespin on the clit. (Not recommended!) But on the labia, clothespins feels kind of nice, almost like having balls.

They're also commonly used in cock and ball torture (which we'll get into later). You can fit a surprising amount of them on a penis and a set of testes. And, much like spanking, clothespins provide an economical kink.

Always note that the less skin you capture within the clothespins, the more painful the experience is going to be. Larger amounts of skin in the clamps is less painful. And when you do take them off, do it *slowly*. Having once had a clothespin ripped off my clit at warp speed, I am very serious about this last point.

For example . . .

A Japanese businessman who Annie and I used to see together invented one of my favorite S&M clothespin-related games. The three of us had rented a dungeon space for this particular session because Annie had a houseguest staying at the Chelsea who likely would not have appreciated our game.

Anyway, this gentleman led Annie and me to the doorway, which led to the "library," which was actually a fake library because it was filled with whips and chains and books—which no one ever read—and was much like the fake schoolroom I used in other sessions. He put wrist and ankle cuffs on Annie and attached her wrists to eyehooks at the top of the doorway. Her ankles, he attached to hooks at the bottom of the doorway.

"This is my favorite position," Annie giggled.

Producing two wooden clothespins, he attached them to the skin just above her armpits. He then took two plastic clothespins with little silver weights on the ends of them and attached them to her labia. As mentioned above, while this sounds painful, it is not. However any type of clamp, clip, or weight on the clit is excruciating.

Annie looked down at the weights and said, "So, this is what it's like to have balls." (Though let's be honest, Annie had "balls.")

He then took out a set of nipple clamps and attached them to her nipples.

"Okay," he said, turning to me. "Now we are going to play a game. I'm going to blindfold you, and you are going to remove these with your mouth." He gestured to the clothespins, "Start here and work your way down."

He slipped the blindfold over my eyes. Moving my tongue gently across her body, I found the first clothespin. It reminded me of the game Operation, and I thought about how greed is the central theme of all games. A friend of mine once pointed out that most children's games can be summed up as, "You get all your things, you put 'em in your thing, and then you win!"

Yet Another Thing You Can Do with Clothespins

The same Japanese businessman I spoke of did another session with Annie and me where clothespins served a different purpose. (If this book were a yoga class, this would be an "advanced" exercise, so please don't try at home till you have more experience. This should give you a good idea of the scope of possibilities clothespins, ingenuity, and a couple of mousetraps can provide.)

I was about to be "tortured" for some imaginary transgression and was lying prone on a small, leather table, which they scooted under a doorway whereupon they cuffed my wrists and ankles to the table's shackles. Annie then unexpectedly pulled two mousetraps out of her bag of tricks. These she clamped to my nipples. She then tied the mousetraps together using a long piece of yellow string, which she tied to an eyehook at the top of the doorway. This made the mousetraps stand erect so that anytime anyone so much as grazed the string, it sent waves of pain through my upper body.

Stranger still, Annie pulled out two plastic, yellow, monkey-shaped clothespins. These she attached to my labia, which didn't hurt at all. It was actually quite pleasant, but then she tied the little monkeys together using another piece of yellow string, which she attached to the eyehook at the top of the door.

The businessman then attempted to put wooden clothespins on the flesh above my armpits. This was my limit. After a second, I screamed my safe word "Mercy!" and he removed them.

Once I was in this position—nipples attached to mousetraps attached to string attached to the top of the door frame, which was also attached to yellow, monkey clothespins attached to my labia—they began to tickle me while bringing me to a big O with a Magic Wand.

And S&M is like a board game with human game pieces. I removed each clamp and clip deftly. If this were an Olympic event, I'd be a gold medalist. She breathed a sigh of relief each time I removed another piece. When I got down to the final pieces, I let my tongue linger before removing them. I handed him the final piece with my mouth.

Okay, so that's a lot to digest. If you are with a new partner, only do one or two things at a time, maybe tickling and clothespins. Then slowly work your way up to the potpourri of kinks described.

Taste—Everybody loves food and, with sensation play, you can eat! (Cuz, you know, *taste* is a sense . . .) You can blindfold your lover and feed your partner while fondling him or her. Maybe make your partner smell each food item and try to guess what it is. If your lover's not diabetic, buy a bag of jelly beans and have him or her sniff and guess the flavor of each one before feeding them to him or her. Make sure you are aware of any food allergies your lover has because the last thing you want is his or her face expanding like a balloon. Otherwise, playing with food, like a Hungry Man dinner, is certain to satisfy your craving.

Smell—The human olfactory system is complicated *and* it goes hand-in-hand with food. Otherwise, the smell and taste of a Madeleine cake wouldn't have lit a fire under Proust's ass to churn out 1.5 million words. Blindfold your love and (as you would with the food activity above) wave an array of scents under your partner's schnozz— essential oils, flowers, or other enticingly fragranced items. If you are using flowers, maybe even get crazy romantic and make a bed of them. (Just because you're getting kinky doesn't mean you also can't be romantic.)

Touch—Obviously, we've been talking about touch a lot here—almost a touch too much. Spanking, paddling, hot wax, caning . . . it's all part of touch. However, touch is strangely often overlooked.

As mentioned earlier (when I spoke of Dick School) we are all so caught up in our heads that we sometimes forget we have bodies. Sensory play should *remind* you that you have a body, that *skin* is your largest organ. People put down skin all the time with phrases like "only skin deep," and yet they spend thousands trying to preserve said skin instead of just enjoying the hell out of it.

To get back in touch with your body, take a break from some of the kinkier stuff described herein and try this fun activity I used to do with patients at Dick School: Recline with your partner totally naked, eyes closed. Take your partner's hand and loosely guide it over your body (except for the genitals . . . too distracting), giving a "tour" of all the places you liked to be touched. You will undoubtedly discover new places you like to be touched. Do this wordlessly and once you are done, reverse roles.

Often we followed this up with another wacky little exercise called Object Game. In Object Game, I picked out three objects (nothing sharp or dangerous) and placed each item, one at a time, on the patient's penis. The patient, whose eyes were closed, then had to describe the temperature, texture, and shape of each object. This was to teach him to focus on penile sensation. I remember placing a tissue over the penis of a patient and him telling me it felt like "the dress of a little fairy."

Both the body tours game and Object Game involved gentle touch, which isn't something that gets spoken about much in BDSM, but I can't stress the importance of it enough. When your sub is tied up, caress her, kiss her, and show her love. Appreciate the skin he or she is in and the skin you are in. If you flog someone's ass, take time to massage that ass. If you are a sub, speak up and ask for that ass massage if you want it.

Now once you've shown each other lots of love, there are plenty of implements you can bust out that will bring great pleasure in the touch-too-much department. My fave raves include:

The Wartenberg Wheel—This is the amazing little pinwheel I described earlier. *Gently* roll it over your partner's skin and watch all his or her hairs stand on end (along with everything else).

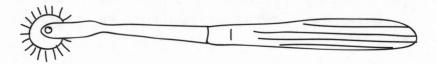

Feathers—The least complex of all BDSM toys? I'd say so. Basically you just run them up and down your partner's bodacious body ostensibly. There are plenty of great cat toys with feathers on them that you can use to tickle and tantalize your lover while he or she is blindfolded or bound.

And speaking of human bondage, I think it's time we finally covered this incredibly important aspect of BDSM. . . .

Human Bondage!

When it came to writing the all-important bondage chapter, I had no idea where to begin. I have spent most of my time being *tied up*, not doing the tying. In fact, aside from my dungeon experience, for four years I played a superhero on a cable access show called *The Adventures of Electra Elf*. As Electra Elf, I was tied up in pretty much every episode but, again, never did much tying up myself.

I suck at tying knots. I can barely tie my shoelaces, which I rarely ever do anyway because I mostly wear go-go boots. For me, writing a chapter on bondage is like not going to law school and then cramming for the bar exam in a week. But I knew that amongst my cavalcade of wacky friends, at least one would be willing to help me with the daunting task of explaining bondage to others. Luckily, I found plenty of help and advice.

One thing about bondage—it is more than simply tying someone up. While it can be defined as "the tying, binding, or restraining of a person for the sexual, aesthetic and/or psychological pleasure of the parties involved," there is more to it than technique. My friend Scooter admitted that, like me, she's not so great at tying people up, but she's superb at "mental bondage."

"I'll just say 'Don't move until I tell you to' and it works," she said. Mental bondage is a great way to start out down this debauched road. It could be as simple as making your sub just stand in the corner with his eyes closed, then slowly caressing him when you are damn good and ready. One step further—incorporating a bit of physical restraint— could also be as simple as pinning a lover's arms down and telling him not to move while you give him head. (I had a lover do this to me once and we almost drowned in female ejaculate.)

Chains, Whips, and Cuffs

In this section, we'll cover everything from mental bondage to rope bondage and orgasm control. Bondage may be used as an end unto itself or it may be used as a part of steamy sex *or* it might even be used in a public party or club scene. Being an attention whore, I naturally enjoy all three from a submissive's perspective. Even during my graduation from Princess Reform School, when I was naked, blindfolded, and tied to a wooden X (in a room that I was certain contained everyone from the mailman, to the video store hipster, to my junior high school guidance counselor) and random partygoers came and went, occasionally commenting upon or caressing my bound, half-naked presence, I enjoyed the attention being lavished upon me. So if the sub gets attention and, hopefully, sexual or psychological pleasure . . . what does the Dom get out of it?

I asked Amanda Whip, Mr. Hall, and Scooter Pie, "Why bind someone?" They offered a number of reasons. Like most BDSM activities, the trust and communication involved in bondage can bring two people together. Plus, it's the ultimate power exchange. For the Dom, you feel that you can do "anything" to the helpless sub at your mercy. (Of course, you can only if it's consensual.) Scooter said, "It's fun to tie them up and entice them to *want* to move."

Everyone agreed that while a sub is bound, especially when her legs are spread wide open, it's fun to "kiss up and down her body" before finally diving in and giving her oral whereupon the Dom can exercise "orgasm control." Though not *technically* part of bondage, I'll discuss orgasm control later along with several other bondage-related activities for novices.

Before any scene involving bondage, the partners should decide, what—if anything—will happen to the sub when he or she is bound. Do you want to tie the sub's ankles together before taking her from behind? Do you want to tie her spread-eagle to the bed before taking her from the front? Or do you just want to tie him up because it looks cool?

Bondage is not always sexual. I had plenty of clients who just liked to tie me up and look at their handiwork. When done well, bondage is an art form. If you want to learn more than the limited instructions this one section can provide, I can't recommend *The Seductive Art of Japanese Bondage* by Midori enough.

But reading isn't enough. Get some rope and practice, practice, practice—and always be safe. When it comes to learning more complex methods of bondage, the best learning technique is hands-on and face-to-face with someone who already knows what he or she is doing.

If you and your partner have just been introduced to the world of bondage, remember these very basic safety precautions:

- Remember that safe word!
- Never leaving a bound person alone. (This includes not practicing "self-bondage" alone in case of an emergency. At the very least, make sure your roommate is home, not wearing headphones, and also not tied up in case your house catches fire or something. A good rule of thumb with bondage is "never get yourself into something you can't get out of.")
- Avoid positions or restraints that may induce postural asphyxia, which occurs when someone's position prevents them from breathing adequately. When that position is the result of the use of restraint, the legal term that is now used is "restraint-related positional asphyxia." A chillingly significant number of people die suddenly during restraint by police, correctional officers, and medical staff. (Sorry, this book just took a not-so-fun turn, but before you decide to hogtie your heifer or sissy boy, know the facts!)

  Research has suggested that restraining a person in a face-down position is likely to cause greater restriction of breathing than restraining a person face up. Trauma can be prevented. One of the most important things a Dom can do is frequently ask, "Are you okay?" If the sub's hands or feet are tingling or numb at all, get him or her out of bondage ASAP. Clearly, if his or her

---

hands look bluish, move as fast as you can to get him or her out of whatever position he or she is in (though it should never get to this point with proper care).

- Make sure the sub changes positions frequently.
- Be certain the restraints are not too tight.
- Do not place rope across the front of the neck.
- Have a PAIR OF SCISSORS on hand.

This last point is not to be overlooked. I recall fooling around with a sound guy in the office of a bar where I'd just performed when he suddenly ripped my fishnet stockings off, tied my wrists together behind my back with them, and went down on me. This was fun and hot, but after I reached orgasm (about two minutes in), we realized we couldn't untie the fishnets. It was as if they'd been soldered together. (It's best to avoid pantyhose and scarves as restraint devices for this very reason. If the sub pulls against them the knots can get drawn too tightly to untie.) But I was hardly thinking straight and I was in no position to look for a pair of scissors, so the sound guy frantically rooted through the desk drawers and came up with nothing. Finally, he bravely (and pantslessly) wandered out to the bar where a helpful bartender gave him a pair of scissors.

Don't be an idiot like I was.

As mentioned before, learning from an experienced partner face-to-face is the best way to "learn the ropes" of bondage. I therefore asked my friend, Stormy Leather, to come over and help me with this section. Stormy is a burlesque performer, go-go dancer, and model who often incorporates self-bondage into her onstage routine. She agreed to show me how to tie myself up. I figured this would be handy once I'd effectively alienated everyone else in my life. As it turns out, tying yourself up is even harder than tying someone else up and, as I already pointed out, you should never practice self-bondage you can't get out of alone.

When Stormy arrived at my apartment, she brought several varieties of rope with her. My favorite was a $\frac{5}{16}$ of an inch thick, Pepto Bismol® pink

30-foot coil of soft nylon. She also brought along twisted hemp rope, the most traditional of the Japanese bondage ropes. I love hemp, but not so much on my skin. It feels a bit too scratchy, like hay.

However, when it comes to bondage rope, it all boils down to personal preference. You'll often hear people say they find nylon too slippery and prefer hemp or cotton. To each his own. Stormy had procured her rope at Purple Passion, one of New York's premiere BDSM supply stores. If you live in Idaho and still want bright pink nylon rope, you can conveniently get it at their website: www.purplepassion.com. Of course, you can always get "not pink" rope at hardware stores, which I generally avoid because (at least in my 'hood) the employees are condescending, machismo shitheads towards women and I don't need memories of their faces flashing before me as I am tied up and taking it in my love-hole.

Anyway, Mr. Hall arrived shortly after Stormy did, carrying cotton rope ($\frac{1}{4}$ of an inch which he'd gotten at the hardware store and had then attached to a pair of restraints). My apartment is sort of like downtown New York's version of Mr. Roger's home only all the people who just "stop by" are usually kooky artists up to something deviant or creative.

Getting back to Mr. Hall's restraints and rope, restraints really are a bondage enthusiast's best friend. They are easy to use and visually appealing, so let's start with them before we get into Stormy's tutorial on rope bondage. FYI—When it comes to *physical* bondage, three main devices are generally used: restraints, handcuffs, and rope. But nowadays with the advent of BDSM web superstores, you can find some incredible bondage kits that come with fancier items like spreader bars, slings, connecting chains, and collars, but let's keep it simple for now.

Types of Restraints

Bondage Restraints (Leather or Pleather Cuffs)—Cuffs are generally comfy so the sub can focus more on what the Dom is doing and less on whether rope or metal handcuffs are digging into the skin too tightly. Meanwhile, the Dom can focus on being sensually dominant rather than on being MacGyver or a rope-tying expert. The great thing about "made for BDSM" cuffs is that they are quick and easy to put on and take off. When they have soft padding or fleece on the inside, they are less likely to bruise or chafe.

The ones Mr. Hall brought over were leather with a padded interior and five eyelets for tightness adjustment. They also had small metal D rings on the sides, which he could attach the rope to and then ostensibly attach the rope to a bed or to a pair of matching ankle cuffs or even to the spreader bar the cuffs apparently came with. And, as Mr. Hall explained, one should not let the décor of his or her home dictate how the cuffs are used. You can screw an eyehook into the ceiling and attach a very long piece of rope to it. Then you can attach the rope to the cuffs. When "normals" come over, you can hide the cuffs and just hang a plant from the hook.

Handcuffs—Maybe it's my fear of the po-po, but conventional handcuffs frighten me. Also, since I lose my apartment keys, my phone, and my charger daily, I have a very real fear of losing the keys to whatever handcuffs I might procure.

Unlike bondage cuffs, the primary goal of handcuffs is not comfort and safety, but immobilization and prevention of escape, so they are not padded to reduce the risk of nerve damage and other injuries. Metal can also hurt skin tissue or cut off the blood circulation if the handcuffs get locked too tightly, so be extra careful with them and make sure you have an extra set of keys or a locksmith's number close at hand. (I smell a porn plot a-brewing . . . "Did somebody call a locksmith?")

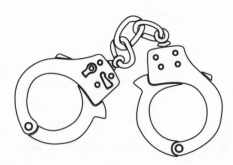

Because of safety concerns, I would only recommend metal cuffs for light play and shorter sessions and *only* double-locking cuffs where the setting that it is already on won't change. You don't want cuffs suddenly getting tighter and causing nerve damage. Just know that when metal cuffs are used, bruising is always a possibility. If you've ever been arrested at a protest, you know this all too well!

Rope Bondage—Rope bondage really deserves its own book . . . one that I am unfit to write. Luckily, there are many books out there specifically devoted to it. There are also many pros and cons to rope bondage. On the one hand, it looks pretty when done expertly and, on the other hand, like a well-executed work of art, it's not easy to do.

Rope is inexpensive, easy to obtain, and easy to store—not like having a giant fuck swing in your kitchen. Remember, your knots don't have to be perfect. After all, little in sex *is* ever perfect. Still, you will find many "rope experts" online giving complex instructions that will baffle anyone who has never been a scout, a sailor, or into the outdoors in any way, shape, or form (me).

Make Your Own Rope Handcuffs

1. Start by making two loops in your rope, each about 10 inches long.
2. Cross the left loop over the right, creating a third loop in the center.
3. Thread the loop that is now on the right through the new center loop, creating a knot.
4. Pull the knot taut before placing your partner's hands though the loops to make "cuffs."

If I was able to figure this out, you will be able to, too. And I'm sure if I didn't have two jobs and a wild rope-obsessed kitten attacking me as I attempted to learn rope bondage, I would be excellent at it.

For example . . .

Speaking of my rope-obsessed kitten, he immediately took a shine to Stormy's rope when she visited to help me with this section. My kitten attacked the robe as she stripped down to a thong. "Do you have a thong?" Stormy asked me. "It's much easier to do this in a thong." I rifled through my underwear drawer, knowing there was not a single thong to be had.

"Nope. It's only granny panties," I told her.

"That's cool. I brought you an extra," she said, pulling out what appeared to be a size zero piece of fabric, barely visible without a monocle.

"Is that Garanimals brand? Will it cut my circulation off before we even get to the rope?" I asked.

"Just put it on!" she said, clearly annoyed at her new pupil.

Soon we were both naked except for our thongs and each holding 30-foot coils of nylon rope. She got to keep the pink and I was given blue. We were about to do a Partial Tortoise Shell Body Harness (Kikkou). I don't know why I felt it imperative to be overly ambitious for the sake of literature, except that the Tortoise Shell looks cool and isn't too restrictive on the body. Plus it creates anchor points for other positions.

In the end, I found it wasn't terribly difficult to execute because I had a hands-on instructor. This is why I would highly suggest attending a workshop on rope bondage if it's something you really want to get into. It's like learning to drive—much easier to get behind the wheel with someone in the passenger seat who has a license.

We started by smoothing out our rope. You should always do this to make sure there's no detritus hanging off it, like preparing for a space shuttle launch. We then folded our respective coils of rope in half and each placed the center point on the spine at the back of our necks while the rest of the rope dropped over our shoulders and breasts.

"It's cold!" I noted, as my magic wands stood erect upon coming into contact with the rope.

Meanwhile, Stormy was battling to keep the kitten away from her new pink rope. "Back off, you!" she said as he leapt into the air, apparently as excited about bondage as I was.

We then brought the two lines of rope into the center of our chests near the sternum (far from the neck!) and tied them in a simple overhand knot. Letting the rope drop farther, we then tied another simple knot between our teats and yet another just below the belly button. We then bent down slightly and pulled the rope slightly apart and under our thong-clad vulvas. Now I could see why Stormy suggested I do the exercise in a thong instead of my pajamas. It felt good! But as we looped the rope behind us, she warned, "Don't pull it too tight or you'll get a cameltoe nightmare!"

We then wove the rope from back to front, in a tortoise shell pattern. This is where practice makes perfect and I doubt I would have been able to do it without Stormy's help. It is impossible to see what you are doing in the back, so you just have to feel for the rope. However, once the mission was complete and we were both fully decorated like Yertle the Turtles with boobs, I could see the appeal of the Tortoise Shell Body Harness. It accentuates the human form and the rope teases many erogenous zones. It's also not too tight and doesn't limit mobility, though Stormy demonstrated how a Dom might tug on the back of the harness while he or she is "having her way" with you. Apparently this harness is also used in suspension, but this is a BDSM book for beginners and I don't want anyone falling from the ceiling.

Rather than continue on about rope bondage, I can only suggest again that you practice different combos and make safety your main concern. In the beginning, keep it simple.

Moving on, let's discuss something that can be done while a sub is restrained with rope, cuffs, or even a simple verbal command: the "Tie and Tease."

Orgasm Control—*Erotic sexual denial,* also known as orgasm denial, is a sexual practice in which a heightened state of arousal is maintained for an extended length of time without orgasm. This sometimes involves long-term denial and the use of chastity belts. This sounds like a living hell to me, so instead we are going to discuss *orgasm control*, a process that requires a sub to ask a Dom for permission to come. Often this is done while the sub is tied up and teased with, say, a vibrator or the Dom's tongue. The sub must then ask the Dom, "Can I come yet, Master?" And the Dom can respond yea or nay.

Orgasm control is almost the opposite of what everybody else on Earth is trying to do: shoot loads across the room. (If you've ever gotten spam mail, you know this appears to be a worldwide goal.) With orgasm control, the idea is to keep your sub on the brink until he or she is near a state of lunacy.

For example . . .

While vacationing with my aforementioned go-go boots-loving British lover, I'd been caught using the water jets in the hot tub "inappropriately" and was immediately taken up to the hotel room, stripped of my bikini, bound, and fucked. Orgasm control had become a big part of our repertoire. Note how we had fun with it:

"Now, young lady, I'm not sure you should be allowed to come," he said, thrusting into me. "You were such a dirty girl downstairs."

"What if I beg you?"

"That might just do the trick."

"There's going to be a lot of begging."

"God, you have the filthiest mind and the wettest pussy I have ever known."

I tried to contain my orgasm as I muttered the word "please" several times until he finally said "yes," whereupon I immediately begged for a second orgasm.

"Can I please come again?" I asked.

"Oh, yes. You can do anything you like," he said, coming close to his own orgasm.

I pulled him closer and came again, contracting tightly around him. As he came, he noticed the Bible on the nightstand.

"Oh, Merciful Lord in Heaven . . . I think I've found God!" he exclaimed, exploding inside of a condom while plucking the good book from the nightstand. "Oh dear Jesus," he said again, falling on top of me.

We convulsed with laughter as he held the book in the air.

"Get that thing away from me!" I screeched.

"Not until you've stopped all your sinning."

"No chance in that."

During this episode, I was loosely tied up and could have easily pulled a Houdini, slipping out of the knots, but the fun was *psychological*—pretending to be the damsel in distress. (Though I was hardly kidding about my commitment to "sinning.")

What if simple pretending, cuffing, and light binding aren't quite enough? Perhaps, you want to be completely bound or you want to completely bind another? There is always mummification.

Mummification—Just a touch more elaborate than all the above, this practice involves restraining a living person's body by wrapping it head to toe or neck to toe so he or she looks like a mummy! For the millionth time in this book, I'll be perfectly honest here: Though I have great interest in ancient Egyptian art and even went so far as to build giant Isis wings, paint myself gold, and go nude (except for the wings and a pair of gold panties) to a party, I have never made anyone up to look like a mummy, not even on Halloween. But apparently mummification is a popular form of sensation play and bondage.

Usually the body wrapping is done with materials like plastic wrap, cloth, bandages, duct tape, body bags, or straightjackets. Those who like to be mummified describe it as an almost transcendent experience, like being in a sensory deprivation tank. As with most forms of bondage, watch for circulation problems and be especially careful to keep all wrapping materials away from the subject's face to prevent breathing restriction accidents.

Obviously, this is not a one-person job and were I ever to be mummified, I would want to do it at some sort of fetish event where there are plenty of people around and someone standing nearby with surgical safety scissors. Never mummify yourself alone. (I didn't think this was even possible, but having now watched innumerable mummification videos online, it appears it is.)

It also appears some of these mummies like to have holes strategically cut in their "wrapping" whereupon some of their parts magically spring to life!

So I have this friend . . .

Actually, my friend, Kat, claims to have had a friend named "Midge" who was not only into eggplant butt plugs (not a good idea), but he would also top it off with head-to-toe mummification with silver duct tape and just a couple of air holes for his nose and mouth. She reports that there was a lot of patchy, red, swollen skin in the aftermath. Kat also mentioned that Midge had a hook in his closet, which he hung from while "duc't up."

Please don't try what Midge did at home.

Spreader Bars—Say you want to be suspended like Midge, just not in a closet while mummified? What are your options? If you have the money, renting out space in a commercial dungeon will provide you with fancy crank-operated suspension bars and lots of other fun equipment. However, if you are on a budget like most regular folk, it need not interfere in the fulfillment of your wildest, kinkiest dreams.

It is possible to suspend a loved one (or vice versa) at home using a simple spreader bar and the aforementioned eyehook in the ceiling. (Just make sure it's been sturdily installed. Mr. Hall recommends attaching said hook to a support beam and asking your hardware store person for a hook and chain that will hold fifty pounds more than your play partner.) What's more, a spreader bar can be used for more than just suspension. But what exactly is a spreader bar?

A *spreader bar* is simply a bar made of metal, wood, bamboo, or any other durable material with attachment points for cuffs at each end that can be fastened to wrists, ankles, or knees to hold them apart. A variant of the spreader bar is a simple bamboo rod, used in rope bondage to place your sub in elegant yet sexually available positions regardless of the gender of the bottom. If you're feeling crafty, it's easy to make a spreader bar with a wooden dowel, eyehooks, and basic tools.

Spreader bars are most often used on the ankles either to keep a sub in a spread eagle position or bent over and unable to do much else (except, you know, be spread eagle or bent over . . .). Just keep the sub steady so he or she doesn't fall over and make sure the legs aren't spread too far apart for too long because pulled muscles are a bitch, as is waking up to your beloved sub screaming from charley horse pains at four in the morning.

A Coffee Table—Bet ya didn't think of this one? Me neither. Mr. Hall, "the Bob Vila of BDSM," did. When you live in small New York City studio apartments, it pays to be creative. As Mr. Hall pointed out, "A coffee table can provide excellent home décor with a secret purpose. Add some O hooks hidden underneath and you can easily bind your partner/lover/sub to it." This *is* a great idea, but I would recommend against doing this on a *glass* coffee table.

Sex Swings—In the olden days of yore, it was difficult to obtain these complex contraptions, but nowadays, with the advent of the World Wide Web, people order sex swings off of Amazon like they are going out of style. As the UPS man or woman carries the generic package to your door, he or she will have no idea what a kinky fuck you are. The carrier will just think you are having a heavy pair of shoes or a box set of PBS Masterpiece Classic DVDs delivered to your door. Meanwhile, you will revel in the secret knowledge that within a few hours, either you or your partner will be strapped in for the ride of your/his/her life.

While sex swings are not exclusive to bondage or BDSM play, they do involve one partner being bound to a device (the swing) while the other moves about freely. It should be noted that not all sex swings are used to fulfill kinky desires. Individuals with muscular weakness or arthritis use them simply to enjoy sexual activity without undue strain on their weak muscles.

Miscellaneous Gear—Not everyone wants to turn their home into a dungeon, but if you *do*, there are boatloads of opportunities to do so, given the variety of bondage furniture that's out there. There are cages both big and small, made for sleeping, standing, or kneeling. Some are shaped like puppy cages and some like birdcages. Or for several hundred dollars, one can obtain a Renaissance faire-style stockade, a St. Andrew's cross, a spanking horse, or a bondage bench! Even better, some people have garages, tools, and woodworking skills with which to make their own. Of course, all of these things take up space and cost money.

If you are new to bondage . . .

Have a discussion with your partner and ask each other a few simple questions before beginning to establish the scenario:

1. Who will be the Top and who will be the bottom?
2. How will the bottom be bound?
3. What equipment will you need to do this binding properly and safely?
4. Finally, what will transpire once the bottom is bound?

Now we'll move on to a subject not far removed from bondage: collars. They are the Holy Grail of BDSM (except much easier to find).

Collars

Collars are like deviled eggs. People either love them or hate them. Velocity, for instance, hates them. "I can't even stand to wear a turtleneck," she told me. "Or a choker or even have my head up against a pillow case." Personally, I love rockin' a collar out of the sheer narcissistic thrill that comes from knowing *others* enjoy the way collars look. Plus, thanks to visionary fashion designer Vivienne Westwood, what greater punk rock accessory is there than the spiked dog collar?

The "collar as accessory" look has since been adopted by Goths, Steampunks, and, when glowing, by Ravers. *Teen Vogue* (yes, I have a subscription) just featured an article titled "10 Ways to Wear Cute Collars." But in the end, Ms. Westwood said it best: "Fashion is about eventually becoming naked."

What do you put on that others will want to take off? Or, what do you put on that others will want to *leave* on while he or she takes everything else off you? With fans of BDSM, a collar is often the answer.

Whether it's assless chaps or a bikini showing off your best features, everyone likes to be admired. Collars are a great way to show off an elegant, swanlike neck and feminine clavicle. When a collar is worn on a dude, there is an appeal to seeing the "stronger sex" reduced to a pet (or if you have a gladiator getup fetish, that's also quite appealing).

Unfortunately, when I sat down with my friends to discuss collars and innocently made the deviled egg reference, all anyone could talk about was deviled eggs. Few foods manage to stir up the kind of emotion exhibited upon the mention of deviled eggs. This seemingly benign finger food stirs up more impassioned debates than foie gras and veal combined. There are no deviled egg converts. The taste for them is not an acquired taste, something you can grow into or accept into your palate later in life. Whatever your first opinion of deviled eggs is, it's an opinion you will take to your grave and you will disrupt even a BDSM collar-related discussion to go into great, gory detail about the sensory experience of eating one in an attempt to horrify any D.E. hater standing within earshot.

"This is not *Fifty Shades of Deviled Eggs* people! Please focus on *collars*!" I announced to the rabblerousing crowd of weirdos in my apartment (Stormy, Mr. Hall, Scooter, and Velocity). For the record, I hate deviled eggs.

The general consensus amongst the collar-haters in the room is that they felt "choked" wearing them. My only real issue with collars is that when they are too big, they make it look like I'm being treated for whiplash. (Again, I just wanna look pretty!)

But Mr. Hall made a very important point about BDSM collars (as opposed to collars as accessories) and that is that they are a symbolic gesture of submission. A sub who wears a collar to symbolize his or her relationship with another is said to be "collared." Some people conduct formal "collaring ceremonies," which are almost like BDSM wedding ceremonies wherein the collar is much like a wedding ring (but cheaper and without the hassle of a 50 percent divorce rate).

Most BDSM collars are made of black leather and have metal D rings or O rings attached to them. (And by O ring, I don't mean "asshole," but rather the bit of metal hardware shaped like an "O." Just so we're on the same page . . .) This makes it easy to leash your sub and take your partner for a walk even if it's just a walk around the bedroom or a tug in the direction of your crotch. It's never wise to chain the sub's collar to anything if it's overhead and *especially* if the sub is wearing high heels or has poor balance. Also make sure the collar isn't too tight.

In serious BDSM circles, there is strict etiquette revolving around the collar issue. They insist that collars be "locking" and that no Dom should wear a collar even as an accessory. Many "old school" BDSM folks' asses are chapped by the abundance of flimsy collars with Velcro snaps out there and vanilla teens running around in studded collars they just bought at Hot Topic. If you've devoted many years to a Master/slave (Can I Just Have a Sandwich?) relationship, I can see how this might irritate, but the fact is BDSM is becoming more mainstream every day, so not everyone is going to know "the rules," much like I don't know "the rules" for "capturing the heart of Mr. Right."

Also, I find the idea that people have to be in a "partnership" to enjoy collars somewhat limiting. Not everybody is prepared to make the commitment. Some people just wanna wear collars, damn it!

"Professionally," I spent many an hour on my hands and knees being led by leash to whatever throne or ottoman my Master (for that particular session) chose to sit upon. Not exactly something to put on my résumé, but it was often erotic to step down from the lofty pedestal where many a dude hath placed me. Despite my enjoyment of this scenario, I have never been a "collared slave." My nature is just too rebellious.

But never say "never." If I've learned anything doing sex work, performance art, and everything in between, it's to expect the unexpected—even from myself. Maybe in another forty years I'll be sporting a collar at the nursing home.

For the time being, the only collars I've worn have been *play collars*, a generic term for collars used during BDSM activity and not necessarily to display being committed to someone else. These collars only stay on for as long as the activity continues.

Collaring in Master/slave Relationships

In serious BDSM Master/slave relationships, there are different stages of collaring—sort of like the different stages of dating without the tedious "dating" part. Not all Dom/sub relationships are the same, and obviously collars are going to have different meanings to different people.

Chains, Whips, and Cuffs

There are generic terms used to describe the collars involved in the three main stages of a Master/slave relationship. They are:

1. **Collars of Consideration**—This is the "getting to know you" phase collar. It doesn't have to be fancy, maybe a step above what they sell at Petco if you want to impress your sub, but it's more a gesture of courtship. If you are the sub, it's kind of like wearing someone's letterman jacket in high school. It sends a signal to the rest of the crowd that you are taken.

2. **Training Collars**—This collar is usually plain, but sturdier than the above. This is where the two partners see how things might work out in a long-term arrangement. Generally it means formal BDSM training sessions have begun wherein the activities I've discussed in previous sections may be employed—bondage, flogging, caning, paddling, intercourse, humiliation, and more!

   This is where the Dom shows what he or she expects from the sub and where both can start to gauge whether it's going to work out. Sometimes this stage can involve living in sin! If you've gotten to this point, both of you likely have chemistry, which is the one thing you can't fake. You can pretend to like someone or even love them, but chemistry is what happens when normally dormant atoms within the genitals and brain spring to life upon meeting someone.

   So once you know you both have chemistry, you now must ask yourselves a few hard questions to save years of misery, wasted emotional energy, and regret. Do you have the same boundaries? How far do you want to go with the "training?" Now is the time to negotiate.

   Other times, a training collar quite simply symbolizes a relationship where the Dom is "training" the sub in a specific area of service like housecleaning or even taking it in the ass. In other instances, a submissive may wear one while being trained by Doms who do not "own" them—sort of like in Story of O when O was trained at Roissy.

Shock Collars

While looking at a million blogs and websites that discuss training collars, I came upon a disturbing, creepy trend: the use of shock collars as "training collars" on humans, mostly women. First and foremost, I would never support the use of a shock collar on a dog, cat, or other four-legged friend and much as I am a misanthrope at times, I would never support their use on a human either.

Sadly, as long as they are legal, idiots and assholes will buy them and use them to replace proper long-term training of their pets. Still other assholes and idiots will use them on people—including children—as a form of "punishment." No human or animal ever deserves to wear one.

---

3. **A Slave Collar**—This is the "real deal" representing the final stage of commitment. For subs it represents their devotion to their Doms, and for the Doms it represents pride in their slaves. For both partners, it can also represent a desire to share each other's lives in a power exchange. Often a "collaring" ceremony is involved. Much like a wedding (again without the divorce rate, hideous bridesmaids' dresses, or annoying relatives in attendance), it is a celebration that friends and other members of the BDSM community often attend though it can also be done in private.

At this level, the collar symbolizes the Dom's commitment to care for the sub and be responsible for him or her. Meanwhile, acceptance of the collar by the sub is an offering of what else? Submission. This collar is supposed to be worn at all times because it symbolizes a 24/7 "sandwich" relationship. It 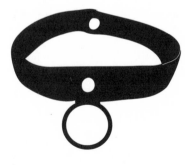 is therefore not always a large leather affair with the word *SLAVE* emblazoned upon it in red. Often it is a simple metal chain and sometimes it is body art—the modern day, kinky equivalent of having your girl's name tattooed on your arm. Many a slave has professed to enjoy sleeping in their collars, especially when enfolded in the protective arms of their Dom. So, if you happen to be out collar-shopping for your sub, consider getting them something as comfy as an old pair of pajamas.

Of course, when it comes to BDSM, the only hard and fast rule that I believe everyone should abide by is "safe, sane, and consensual." As I said in the introduction, let your freak flag fly! Don't be afraid to experiment because if you can't experiment in the BDSM scene, where else are you gonna do it?

Various Other Types of Collars—No Relationship Necessary

There are an infinitesimal amount of collars out there, a few of which aren't even collars at all. Perhaps one of them suits your lifestyle better than the aforementioned traditional set. *Maybe* you don't have a partner and just want to play. *Maybe* you do have a partner, but like my friend, Velocity, you can't even deal with turtlenecks. *Maybe* you just want to announce to the world that you love BDSM. There are many ways to do this . . . I am sure there are ones I have never even heard of.

Ring of O—Much like the ring in *Lord of the Rings*, a Ring of O has great power. I should know because, Annie, my partner in crime at the Chelsea, wore one and she could convince me to do pretty much anything she liked. I felt like Gollum in her presence.

The Ring of O is a specially designed ring that has been worn as a distinctive mark in the BDSM community since the 1990s. The name derives (of course) from the ring worn by O in *Story of O*, though the ring in the novel has a different symbolic meaning than the one worn by BDSM folk today. In the book, the ring is worn by female "slaves" who have finished their training at Roissy and are therefore obliged to be obedient to any man who belongs to the secret society of Roissy. Today, people wear such rings to denote that they are interested in BDSM and to wordlessly share whether they are Tops or bottoms.

Though not a crucial bit of info and probably something you'll never be asked on *Jeopardy*, it should be noted that the ring in the novel is an iron signet ring with a triskelion symbol on the top. It is a Celtic symbol consisting of three legs or lines radiating from the center. The symbol is said to have several meanings including "man's progress" and the circle of life, death, and birth, but I think the "third leg" has a pretty obvious meaning. The modern ring has no triskelion on it, but is rather a simple cylindrical steel ring with a little O ring attached (again, an O-shaped piece of metal, not an asshole).

A Protective Collar—This shows that a Dom is protecting the sub who is wearing the collar. It acts like a safety net when the sub feels uncomfortable in certain social situations. Maybe the sub has been in an abusive relationship and someone is bothering or harassing him or her. This collar basically sends a "lay the fuck off my sub" message to the world. So if a sub is at a club (this sounds like Dr. Seuss!) where old men with tampons up their asses are being crass jackasses, this collar makes a sub feel like he or she is free from bother.

Neck Corsets—Both women and men wear neck corsets—lots of Goth women and men actually. Often they are simply out and about, lookin' cool in fetish clothing. As the name would suggest, a *neck corset* (sometimes called a throat corset or neck lacer) is a type of corset worn fitted around the neck. However, unlike a waist corset, it should be worn loosely to prevent not being able to breathe and, thus, dying.

Cyber Collar—This was bound to happen and many BDSM players aren't happy about it—*the cyber collar*. It is what the Internet has wrought. But given I spend about seventy-five hours a week on Facebook, who am I to judge?

Basically, people meet in specialized chat rooms or on BDSM sites and have cyber Dom/sub relationships. This is a world I will admit to knowing nothing about. What I do know is that I am lucky enough to live in a city full of millions of people where I am part of a creative circle of individuals who are kinky, creative, bohemian, outspoken, artistic, fun, and amazing so I have never searched for a partner on the web.

However, I know there are people who live in say, Alaska, or other less populated areas, who might want to have their cock and balls tortured or their titties clamped and they must be hellishly frustrated. So they find partners on the web! While this might be a cure for loneliness, ennui, and existential angst, it isn't *always* a good idea—and not necessarily for the reasons that seem to piss off so many BDSM practitioners.

I found many bloggers bitching about how "lightly" cyber partners took the "collaring ritual" along with complaints of how so many online subs were "greedily" trolling for as many "cyber collars" as possible. Some bloggers also seemed bothered by the fact that too many vanilla people were invading the turf of lifestyle BDSM practitioners.

While searching the web, I started to feel like *West Side Story* with the vanilla "BDSM curious" people and the "sandwich" people role-playing the Sharks and the Jets. Maybe I have a little too much empathy for the lonely, horny people who get into BDSM antics online, but I have no problem with the vanilla, yet curious, crowd checking out the scene. (In fact, I would consider myself somewhere in between. I can take and enjoy a caning, but don't want to wear a collar to bed . . . at least not yet.)

What I *do* have a problem with is the fact that BDSM involves physical and emotional risks and on the web that risk is doubled. Know *who* you are getting into a chat room with and *what* you are doing. If you do agree to get together with a potential play partner, meet him a few times for some "straight time" in a social setting before you just hand him a flogger and tell him to have at it. But that's pretty much all I can say on the subject because I am not Mark Zuckerberg and I have no power over what you see on the web, hence I will now end this public service announcement and talk to you about fisting.

(By the way, I also have no power over fisting but I can, at least, give you a helping hand . . .)

Fisting the Night Away!

While fisting is not exclusively a BDSM activity and I am sure there are *handfuls* of people who fist the night away without leather, latex, whips, and chains, it *is* a subject worth covering here given it's a taboo kink where one partner is the bottom and one is the Top—or rather one is *in the bottom*. Entire books have been written on the subject of fisting, so if you really want to learn more, wrap your fist around one of them.

Fisting is an intimate act that involves placing or attempting to place the entire hand (or even both hands) in the rectum or vagina. Once the hand is fully inserted, extreme gentleness and patience are required—move it in and out of the orifice at a "slow and low" tempo.

Fisting can be dangerous if not performed correctly.

Fisting can cause laceration or perforation of the vagina, perineum, rectum, or colon, resulting in serious injury and even death. That's why *patience* is the key word here. As Scooter pointed out, "If you think you are going slow, you probably aren't going *slowly enough*." Scooter, by the way, has fisted herself onstage. Admittedly, she has tiny hands.

Having only ever been *vaginally* fisted, I cannot speak for those who've taken it in the ass. I can say, however, that they may be my heroes. And to be honest, I've only been fisted once.

For example ...

It was at the Chelsea and I lay on my back, frightened, while
Annie produced a tube of K-Y. She warmed a generous amount

between her hands and lay beside me. She inserted two fingers in my pussy, followed slowly by a third. Like most lesbians, she had well-trimmed nails. (I don't like to generalize, but most lesbians do have short nails for a reason. That's why mainstream porn featuring girl-on-girl action where both have dagger-long nails is so absurd. When I look at those nails, all I can think is *ouch!*)

There is no way this is going to work, I thought, as Annie moved at a snail's pace and my pussy stretched to what I imagined was its limit. Soon, though, her pinky was inside of my stretched-out vertical smile. After working her first four fingers in, her thumb joined the crowd and I began to sweat profusely. Breathing deeply, I relaxed and was no longer frightened.

I can't say it felt "incredible," but it felt "interesting," which sadly is the least interesting adjective in the English language . . . yet it's all I can come up with to describe the sensation. Amazingly, Annie used her free hand to take a close-up Polaroid of her "handiwork," which is probably floating around in cyberspace right now and will likely surface the moment I am asked to marry into royalty. Luckily, I wouldn't even recognize my vagina in a fisted state so no one else should either.

As I was being fisted, I marveled at how stretchy and durable my vagina is. Given babies emerge from vaginas (with a great deal of effort), this shouldn't have come as a shock. As the very wise Golden Girl Betty White once pointed out, "Why do people say 'grow some balls?' Balls are weak and sensitive. If you wanna be tough, grow a vagina. Those things can take a pounding."

Scooter reiterated this. "Once your hand's inside, it feels fragile, but the vagina is *strong*."

Tips for Better Fisting

Because my nerves were wracked during my one and only experience with fisting, it wasn't exactly a magical moment—more like a surreal one. But I can give a few pointers on fisting, offered by friends and other resources. They are as follows:

- Trim and moisturize your damn nails. No one wants to be fisted by a dry-cuticle-plagued sloth.
- Use lots of lube. Lots.
- Unless you know your partner very well, wear a latex glove.
- Don't *start* with a fist. Start with a finger, then make a little duckbill with your hand.
- Move your hand slower than The Little Engine that Could until you have reached that magical, warm place.
- Unless your fistee starts freakin' out, once you've reached that place, you can form a fist. (If the fistee does freak out and begins to strangulate your hand with either his sphincter muscles or her vag, pull out as slowly as the aforementioned sloth would cross a street.)
- *And* if you are the fistee who starts to freak out, first say your safe word to stop the activity and then breathe slowly into your stomach. Easier said than done, but *relax* as your lover pulls out. You will be okay with these simple precautions.

Into Golden Showers?
Urine Luck!

Now that we've covered fisting, let's talk about pee! A lot of people like to be pissed on . . . probably a lot more than you could ever imagine. Still, others like to do the pissing. I'm not gonna judge. I'll even admit (in this presumably best seller) that I once drank *my own* pee, because, frankly, I want you to buy my book, not kiss me. It was many years ago and (of course) for money. Annie and I were doing a session with a Japanese businessman who wanted to watch me pee in a cup and then drink my own piss.

"No way," I said. Drinking *my own* pee would be less humiliating than drinking *someone else's* pee, but it was just not my cup of tea. My cup of tea was tea, not urine.

"Gandhi drank his own pee," Annie insisted.

"Yeah, but Gandhi drank his own pee because he was trying to stay alive. My situation is hardly that dire."

Somehow, she convinced me to do it (as she did with everything) and moments later I was peeing in a cup and then drinking it. My urine tasted salty, much like my tears. In a blind taste test, I guarantee subjects would be unable to differentiate between the two. In the end, I realized drinking my own pee was far from terrible, which is something no one should ever have to realize.

But getting back to golden showers: Don't be ashamed and don't feel alone. One glance at YouPorn should be enough to convince you that you are not a completely isolated deviant, though I certainly wouldn't bring up water sports on a first date.

But why would anybody be into *pee* of all things? Like so many other activities in this book, part of the arousal comes from breaking cultural taboos. And if you are into being humiliated, what could be more humiliating than being peed on? Perhaps being shat upon?

A Side Note about Brown Showers

We're only going to simply define brown showers here, given it is a far more fringe activity than golden showers. Executing a *brown shower*, if you've managed to put two and two together, requires shitting on another person. Nothing about shit appeals to me, but again, I am not gonna judge. I hate deviled eggs. Some people love them, but do I judge those people? No.

Getting back to *golden* showers, I will leave you with a few bits of advice.

First, be aware of sexually transmitted infections. Pee contains trace amounts of bacteria, so unless you are sure the pisser is clean as a whistle, don't go there—especially if he asks you to drink his pee.

Also, if you are so obsessed with golden or brown showers (or really any of the fetishes and activities that I've described in this book) that it interferes with your work, home life, or life in general, it's time to seek counseling.

That said, if you are gonna go for the gold, do it in the shower; it makes cleanup much easier. Make sure when you are doing it in the shower that you are sober and balanced. Overall, about two-thirds of accidental injuries happen in the bathtub or shower—which makes sense, because they can become slippery. That pisses me off!

Behind Enema Lines!

Since we just got gritty and talked about fisting and pee, and because I also admitted to drinking my own pee, I guess we can move on to enemas. First, why would anyone want to involve enemas in their BDSM play or sex lives?

Enemas are popular for a number of reasons. On a technical level, they clean the ass out, making it fresh and tidy for anal sex, fisting, and butt plugs. My first day working as a P.A. on a porn shoot, the director said, "We need to get enemas!" Turning to me, he asked, "Wanna come?"

As we walked to a Rite Aid, I tried to process this gritty reality of porn.

Finding the laxative aisle, he tossed an economy pack in his shopping basket. "I'm taking no chances. I'm getting a six-pack," he declared, holding them up for all to see. (We were working on an anal film at the time.) Enemas are a great "anal douche." Porn stars frequently use them before heavy-duty anal scenes. Enemas are to a clean asshole as Viagra is to boners.

However, some people just get off on enemas—the feeling of gushing liquid flowing into their asshole and the subsequent Olympic sprint to the bathroom. For a sub, allowing the Dom to administer an enema can make him or her feel vulnerable, desired, erotically humiliated, and completely at the Dom's mercy, whereas the Dom gets to wield power over his sub by controlling this very personal function. Often enemas are used in "medical fetish" scenes where a "nurse" will administer an enema to a "patient."

Whatever your reasons for wanting to incorporate enemas into your BDSM play, follow three simple rules so you don't become Public Enema #1!

Chains, Whips, and Cuffs

1. *Never* sneak up on someone who is tied up and simply shove the enema nozzle up his or her ass. This is a surprise no one wants. Best to give someone an enema when he or she is not tied up, for obvious reasons.

2. Use lukewarm water only. Not sure if it's an urban legend, but the worst dungeon horror story I ever heard involved a newbie Dom who had been improperly trained administering a (literally) boiling hot enema to her client. (She had been told to "heat it up," but took this advice a little too far.) As one can imagine, this did not result in an erotic experience but rather an ambulance, surgery, and quite likely a lawsuit. Conversely, never give someone an ice-cold enema. If the recipient has a weak heart, it can prove fatal.

3. I'm not going to explain the mechanics of enemas, but know how they work before you use one. (Like so many toys, they come with directions.) Disposable, cheapo ones work just fine, though it's a good idea to dump out the chemical solutions found in most and fill them with lukewarm water.

Those seem to be the main rules of enema etiquette. However, my boyfriend (as I was typing this) just added, "Don't put one in your urethra. I saw that happen once in a video." He's probably correct.

Also, AVOID alcohol enemas. People die from them. (Not just college frat kids hazing each other, but older adults who should know better.) If you want to get drunk, do it the old fashioned way: chug beers and listen to Zeppelin. But remember, BDSM play should be done while sober anyway. Beer is an acquired taste and you don't acquire it through your ass.

Glory HOLEllujah!

Home Décor for Pervs

While discussing this book ad nauseam with friends, we began
to discuss how one could "trick out" their home for BDSM play.
We've already heard from Mr. Hall, "the Bob Vila of BDSM," who
suggested the "overhead eyehook/attachment for a suspension bar/
charming plant holder" idea as well as the "coffee table/bondage
table" ideas.

While these are ingenious and funny, the importance of the space where
you conduct your BDSM play cannot be overlooked. You want to set
the mood. A sloppy Dom spells trouble. If he or she can't handle a mop,
how is a Dom gonna handle a flogger on your ass?

We've already discussed using music to increase dopamine levels, but
what about the space? BDSM should be both sultry and theatrical and a
pile of filthy knickers on the floor and a pyramid of empty beer cans and
dirty dishes in the sink don't add up to sultry *or* theatrical. If you are a
Dom, take a cue from my favorite muscular leatherman Mr. Clean® and
keep your space tidy. (He, Arm & Hammer®, and the burly mustachioed
Brawney® Man might be your best friends when it comes to having a
new play partner over.)

It's also important to keep your equipment organized. Mr. Hall keeps
his in what looks like a Tyvek® "cooler" that has a protective seal to
prevent mold and mildew from accumulating on his leather goods.
Make sure you keep your rope and everything else clean and free of
debris.

Consider various factors in your perverse playtime. If bondage is going
to happen, perhaps don't light candles. The last thing you want to do

What Should Be In Your BDSM Starter Kit?
Safety scissors
Condoms
Lube
Bandages
Rope
Lint roller
Alien mask? (Your choice.)

is leave a tied-up lover alone while you battle flames. And if you have a reckless, wild kitten and an elderly Chihuahua who chases him around the house, candles are also not a good idea because they likely will get knocked over. However, there are many other ways to make one's home a kinky love palace, even if you have rambunctious pets and very little space.

Make Your Own Glory Hole

This was Stormy Leather's idea and it's a good one—perfect for party games. "You could use it at parties, and then win a prize when you guess whose penis you've just taken," she suggested. "There could be prizes and stuff."

(FYI: A *glory hole* is a hole in a wall that someone pokes his penis through and another person *on the other side of the wall* receives this penis in some manner, be it in the ass, pussy, or mouth, all the while not knowing *whose* penis it is. Thus, glory holes facilitate anonymous sex.)

I pointed out that since I live in an old tenement where the bathtub is in a closet in my kitchen, it might be fun to carve a glory hole in the door to the closet bathtub.

Mr. Hall examined the door. "I don't know about that door. It has really thick wood. You would have to bevel it for somebody to even get 2 inches of cock through there."

Good point. You want whatever wood you're going to drill through to be thin and soft. Maybe misuse a "beanbag toss game stand" for perverse purposes if you have no time to carve your own.

Other Ways to Set the Scene

- **Black lights and strobe lights.** (Be sure to ask your partner if he or she has epilepsy before installing a strobe light.) Install a Clapper® so that you can "clap on" these lights at anytime. Delightful surprises!

- **Mirrors. Mirrors everywhere!** One of the reasons why mirrors are so popular in BDSM is because they give both parties more than a couple views of what's going on. If a sub is bound facing a large mirror, she can gaze at her countenance and get a narcissistic high *or* she may be bound with her rear to the mirror, giving the Dom two views at once (and the sub no view at all). However, if you live in an earthquake-prone area, careful with mirrored ceilings. There is always reflective paper.

- **Knit your own butt plug cozy!**

- **A cast-iron molded headboard.** Really, any kind of molded headboard is great for bondage enthusiasts. If you don't have one, install a couple of eyehooks to the wall slightly above the bed.

- **Eggplant, duct tape, and a hook in the closet.** (This from Kat's aforementioned friend.) However, I am going to *strongly caution* against putting eggplant in your ass. Later, we'll talk about what *not* to stick in your ass.

- **Scratch-n-sniff wallpaper.** (This would be fun to use with blindfolds.)

- **Plush carpet.** This one I added in because, as a sub, you spend a lot of time crawling around on your hands and knees. It's nice to have some cushion.

These are just a few ideas. The dungeon I worked in had been decorated with great care and ingenuity. Penis-shaped wall hooks held hundreds of coils of rope while human-sized birdcages and leather masks were displayed on mannequin heads. There was a medieval-looking chair with a dildo protruding from the seat, which apparently wasn't enough because the chair could also be operated, by a crank, to shoot from floor to ceiling.

We can't all afford to trick out our pads like this, and most of us wouldn't want to since relatives might actually visit, but a little creativity goes a long way. Really, all you need is a good drill, some eyehooks, and a dirty mind.

Going Pro

Because many of my friends are both poor and perverted, I have been approached several times about how they might "break into the business" (i.e., become a pro Dom or sub). Since it's been so many years since I did it professionally, I tell them that I honestly no longer have connections in the industry. I don't dissuade anyone from doing it, but I don't persuade anyone either.

From a writer's perspective, working in a dungeon offered a gold mine of stories. From a capitalistic perspective, the industry can be a literal gold mine if you work hard at it (which I never did). Possibly, I didn't put in the "hours" because, from a human perspective, it wasn't easy to be so intimate with strangers. Plenty of my clients were extremely lonely people who believed they were forming a deep bond with me when often that bond was one-sided. Despite the fact that *I* was the sub, my maternal instincts usually kicked in and I wanted to take care of these men even when they were whipping my ass. If only Freud could have been a fly on those rotating walls! Of my clients, I have only remained friends with a couple of them. As the dungeon's head Mistress told me when I first started, "It's much different than doing it for love."

She was right. I have been submissive for love, and, as with anything you do for love, it is earth-shatteringly enjoyable. Doing it professionally was a whole different thing. Sometimes, it really sucked.

However, I would never put it down. The pay was great, which meant limited workweek hours, which in turn meant more time to work on my paintings, screenplays, and books. If you are a sexy thang in need of rent money, the decision is in your hands, but make sure you find a *reputable* place where they take every safety precaution possible to ensure that you will be okay.

Remember that you can say NO to anything even when you are being paid to say YES to a lot of crazy shit. Even when money is exchanged, the credo still applies—*safe, sane, and consensual.*

Edge Play

Speaking of *safe, sane, and consensual,* edge play is a term for BDSM activities that push the boundaries of the safe, sane, and consensual creed. Here is where we get to the aforementioned eggplant and other things you should avoid. (Basically, if you find it in the produce section, it is not intended for your ass.)

Edge play may involve the risk of serious harm, permanent damage to your body, or even death. With activities like cutting, barebacking, and blood play, the risk of spreading diseases also increases. Other activities such as breath play (erotic asphyxiation), gun play, knife play, and fire play are all considered edge play, as well. Because this is a BDSM book for beginners, I would guess that none of the above are on your evening's agenda, but I still must stress the importance of the word *sane* in the safe, sane, and consensual credo.

You might think an activity is safe and you and your partner might both consent to it, but please be *sane*. No kink is worth dying over. I've already cautioned against self-bondage and barebacking (fucking without a condom), which I suppose is probably okay if you and your partner have been tested and/or you don't mind the risk of makin' a baby. So let's discuss breath play, as it appears to be one of the most popular forms of edge play out there.

Breath Control (or "Breath Play")

Given that breathing is how we stay alive, breath play terrifies the bejesus out of me—and it should. It is not something I have ever participated in (out of lack of interest on top of the fear of not breathing and thus ceasing to live). Quite simply, *breath play* is the intentional restriction of oxygen to the brain for the purpose of enhancing sexual arousal. This process is known as *autoerotic asphyxiation* when you practice it alone.

Chains, Whips, and Cuffs

Erotic asphyxiation is the term used when you practice breath play with a partner.

The history of this practice dates back to (at least) the early seventeenth century, when it was first used as a treatment for erectile dysfunction. The idea for this most likely came from observers at public hangings noting that males often popped wood that would sometimes remain after they'd been hanged and died. Occasionally, they ejaculated while being hanged. However, in hanging victims, ejaculation occurs after death because of disseminated muscle relaxation, which is different from the mechanism sought by breath play practitioners.

There have been a few high-profile deaths attributed to autoerotic asphyxiation, but I wondered what the actual numbers were. How many people were cutting off their airflow for the sake of getting off? Being naturally curious, and in no way being an expert on this particular subject, I messaged my sister's ex-boyfriend, who is now an EMT worker in a large Southern city, to ask him about it. He messaged back, "You have to call me because I have too many horror stories."

If that one sentence alone doesn't convince you *not* to try breath play, I'm afraid nothing will. Tragically, lonely teenagers often experiment with the practice of autoerotic asphyxiation, and they often end up dead. According to my EMT friend, the family sometimes "sanitizes the scene," and the death is then falsely ruled as suicide. I had read estimates that showed the death rate from this practice to be about a couple hundred a year, but he insisted that because of the "sanitation" factor, the death toll is probably much higher.

If you are dealing with erectile dysfunction, *please* do not resort to autoerotic or erotic asphyxiation. It is rare that a blood flow problem has anything to do with E.D. and hanging yourself from a belt is not the answer. Rather, please look into sex therapy. If you can't afford therapy (who can?), there are excellent books on the subject. You can even find them at the library, so no money spent and no life lost. (I know this because the manbrarian I spoke of earlier used to check these "study materials" out for me when I first became a surrogate.)

154

There are other even more complicated forms of breath play, as the aforementioned Midge could probably tell you, but I will *strongly caution* (as in, please don't fucking do it) against using any device or mask that inhibits airflow—even if you are with someone who considers him/herself an expert.

Choking

Choking is another big form of breath play and is also quite dangerous (given that it's choking and all . . .). As a generally submissive person, I can see the appeal of some big brawny dude wrapping his manacle hands around your neck and "taking your breath away." But the problem is that once he takes your breath away, you die.

So avoid choking scenarios, as there is really no way to do it safely. If you are the Dom in a choking situation, you could spend years in prison (and years hating yourself for having killed someone) and as a sub you could lose your life.

To summarize, don't do it. Even if your partner is Dr. McDreamy and he's spent decades in medical school and is considered the world's greatest surgeon, don't do it. Even if you are dating the fucking reincarnation of Hippocrates, don't do it. Breath play is simply a bad idea. So is fucking without a condom, but plenty of people are *going* to do it.

As a writer, I understand that I don't have much power over what any of you do between the sheets or on the kitchen floor or wherever else you choose to get kinky. In that case, I would suggest using verbal taunts and humiliation to replace the actual physical activity. Your partner may still experience a rush of adrenaline or fear if you say, "I am going to choke the living shit out of you later, you little slut bitch/sissy/whore." The extreme kink factor will not lose its glory and no one will die or go to prison.

Other Stuff You Shouldn't Do

While on the phone with the EMT, I started asking more questions about "commonplace kink gone wrong."

"Just last week we had a couple in their sixties that somehow got a lychee fruit lodged in the woman's vagina," he said. "No idea what made them think it was a good idea."

"What else?"

"Well, lots of vegetables. You know all you have to do is Google 'rectal X-rays' and you'll be dumbfounded. Last week we had a guy with a one-liter bottle of soda up his ass. It was only one-liter, not two-liter mind you . . . I've seen Barbie® dolls up there."

"Wait, because the heads pop off?"

"Yeah. And, during Halloween, forget it. All the stuff people put in their cornucopias . . . goes right in their asses—zucchini, squash, you name it."

The idea that half of America is stuffing their cornucopias up their assholes when they should all be working on their Halloween costumes left me stunned. What would the Great Pumpkin say? He probably couldn't say anything because he'd be lodged in someone's asshole. When there are so many things designed to go *up* the ass (that can be discreetly ordered on the web), this seems like a terrible tragedy.

Other Edge Play Activities

Plenty of the things we've covered such as enemas and golden showers would, in some circles, be considered edge play, but there are more. Piercing, cutting, fire play, knife play, gun play, and branding fall under this category.

Piercing

Piercing refers to a creating a hole in the flesh. Aside from once having my nose pierced, I am a piercing novice. In BDSM, the most common piercing locations are genitals and nipples. I have found a weird astrological phenomenon—an inordinate amount of male Leos have pierced nipples. Being a Leo, I can say this, but I think it's because Leos like to be looked at and piercing your nipples will ensure that people look at them.

For example . . .

A couple of years ago, I went on a date with a male Leo who wore both vampire fangs *and* nipple rings. You wouldn't know this at first glance because he also wore a tweed suit and happened to be a mathematician.

Anyway, he removed his nipple ring before bed and accidentally left it at my apartment, sort of like when Carrie left her panties at Mr. Big's (a "leave-behind" to ensure you will see someone again).

This vampire mathematician was also one of the few seriously submissive men I have ever gone out with and I had fun with it. He was, at the time, "property" of a Dominatrix who had obnoxiously interrupted my open mic (heckling and being disruptive). She obviously wasn't a very good Mistress seeing as how he banged me and left his nipple jewelry on my nightstand. (They're great in bed, by the way—pierced, vampire mathematicians in tweed.)

So, I gave him an assignment. If he wanted to ever see his nipple ring again, he MUST write a brief essay about how he'd had a *fantastic* time on our date and how I was incredibly beautiful, a fine lay, and the host of the greatest open mic in the universe. The essay ended up being hilarious, brilliant, and something that will make me smile for years to come. (Being the Dom is fun sometimes!)

An Assumption about New Orleans

Another odd piercing phenomenon—which may be inaccurate and could possibly anger some residents of New Orleans—is that everyone from that city seems to have their genitals pierced. It would be interesting to do a per capita study. Maybe this should be a question on the next census: *Do you have any piercings?*

In NOLA, Velocity introduced me to a blue-haired transvestite named Joey who claimed to be both an exhibitionist and a lesbian. He commonly went commando under a miniskirt, which he frequently lifted to reveal a penis pierced with a small disco ball. Each time he got aroused, which was often, the disco ball stood at full mast.

One night Joey, Velocity, and I all went to a bar to play pool with two of Joey's friends—a petite redheaded girl with a pixie cut and a long-haired redheaded buxom babe. They attempted to teach me to play pool, but the rules quickly flew out the window when they discovered I wasn't wearing panties. Soon it did not matter whether I was hitting striped or solid just so long as I was bending over in front of them.

Hours later, we stumbled back to the hotel with Joey and the redheads. I sat down on the couch next to the long-haired redhead who began to discuss her clitoral piercing. *Does everyone in New Orleans have their genitals pierced?* I wondered. Apparently so. I think this because moments later, the pixie lifted up her skirt to reveal *her* piercing. I then lifted up my skirt because it seemed the thing to do—and also because Joey already had his hand up it. Eventually the entire group joined in and the long-haired redhead, who'd boasted earlier about her oral prowess, brought me to orgasm with her tongue.

I realize this has little to do with an "edge play" piercing scene, but sometimes I just like to boast about my sexual adventures.

In a "scene," the Dom often does the piercing though sometimes the sub pierces him/herself. No matter who is doing it, an experienced piercer *should* be present to assist. This ain't like drunkenly piercing your ear in junior high, so professional assistance is highly recommended. Sometimes the piercing is not permanent and only lasts for the duration of the play, but sometimes it can be permanent as in . . . you get some sweet gold hoops through the nipples that have your Dom's monograph inscribed in them.

Cutting

In *cutting*, a scalpel or other fine blade is used to make shallow cuts in the top layer of your partner's arm or in your arm (or anywhere else). You may also carve words and symbols. In high school, I remember the badass metalhead girls carved their boyfriend's initials and Iron Maiden logos into their arms. I was never part of that crowd because I was sort of a nerd. Ironically, they are probably happily married with children while I am sitting here in my run-down apartment writing about them and other perverse shit. (They will likely never know that they are literary figures.)

Get Tested!

Since blood is obviously involved in cutting, there is a risk of hepatitis C and HIV. If you must engage in risky blood play, just as I would suggest throwing a raincoat over your one-eyed snake during intercourse, I suggest wearing latex gloves.

And please, *always* get tested whether you are working with blood play or any other type of play. It's free at most clinics and testing is *the* most effective method for stopping the spread of disease. Most clinics offer counseling services, and please know that if you *do* test positive for HIV, it is NOT the end of the road.

In my lifetime, I have seen AIDS viciously take people's lives. I have also seen the introduction of drugs that not only save lives, but also make HIV a manageable disease—more so than diabetes (which *is* actually the fastest-growing disease in this country). So don't be afraid to get tested!

Cutting is closely related to knife play. However, in knife play, the knife is often simply present to instill fear in the sub, providing an extreme sense of helplessness and vulnerability that is a turn-on to some. However, one slip of the knife and your partner could be dead or missing an eye. It is *never* okay to stab someone, even if he or she asks for it. Remember the *sane* part of "safe, sane, consensual"? Maybe just get some press-on nails and scratch the shit out of your lover instead?

Gun play

In terms of gun play, the risks are insanely obvious. Simply having a firearm in the home increases the risk of a violent death. However, if you are determined to achieve the psychological mind-fuck that might come from toying with one of the only things on Earth less dangerous than the A-bomb, then consider the only safe option there is—buying a *realistic-looking* gun and playing with it. (They sell them online, of course.)

Gun play with a *real* gun may lead to an untimely death or spending the rest of your life as a vegetable because you thought it'd be fun to put a gun in your ass/pussy/mouth. You even run the risk of spending the rest of your life behind bars because you put a gun in someone else's orifice and it accidentally went off.

Maybe gun play with a fake gun won't have the same "danger factor," but there is enough danger afloat in the world without bringing guns into the mix. Whatever you do, *don't* take that realistic-looking gun outside or cops will plant many bullets into your person and you will have no defense because you will cease to live.

Fire play

Fire play is yet another form of edge play. Because I have many freak friends who work at the actual freak show (Coney Island USA!), I know people who swallow fire, breathe fire, and juggle fire. I also know they would probably all say the same thing about fire play: Unless you and your partner are both highly trained fire experts, don't get jiggy with fire. And by experts, I mean both of you are trained firefighters and both are in full-on firefighter gear with hoses and extinguishers nearby.

By the way, *fire play* generally refers to placing an accelerant such as alcohol on a person's body, then igniting and quickly extinguishing it.

My suggestion: Don't do it. And if you do, make sure you have renter's insurance because your home could quickly be ablaze.

Therapy and Transcendence

BDSM is never a replacement for therapy. If your problems and issues make life unbearable or if your interest in BDSM has made life unmanageable, it is best to seek counseling. If the nature of your problem is sexual, I recommend finding a certified therapist who specializes in sexual problems.

I know how scary this is for both men and women. While working at the therapy center, I often answered the phones and the nervous quake in the voice of prospective patients upon their initial call was always heartbreaking. When they eventually came in, they realized something: They were not alone. As heartbreaking as their first calls were, it was exhilarating to hear stories or get letters from patients months after they'd graduated that said that they were doing well "on the outside."

Extreme sexual problems and dysfunction aside, BDSM can be a portal to healing. For many people who have been in physically or emotionally abusive relationships or who grew up in abusive households, BDSM offers some hope. And strangely (despite the thousands of safety warnings I've placed throughout the book), the idea that loving Doms who may whip and erotically "torture" them without truly hurting them physically or emotionally may be part of their healing.

To put all of your trust in another, to make yourself vulnerable to him/ her and in turn have your partner take care of you, is a little like playing the "trust falling game" that used to be so popular at summer camp (and probably still is). In this game, one person falls and a circle of people catch him or her. From a submissive perspective, BDSM is letting yourself fall, knowing you'll be caught in the end, and having a huge adrenaline rush along the way.

From a dominant perspective, BDSM offers the joy of knowing that someone is placing their trust in you and adores and honors you. Being dominant can make one feel powerful and God- or Goddess-like. Oddly enough, being submissive can do the same thing.

While working on this book, I spoke to many friends who have found some peace through BDSM. My friend Shannon is now in a happy marriage that involves kink, pizza/movie nights, and other forms of normalcy. Shannon told me how she first found BDSM and it's a great example of how "the scene" can transform one's life.

For example . . .

"In my teens, I was a cutter," Shannon said. "I don't know how I started or where I learned it, but my best friend and I probably encouraged each other to do it since we were both dark and depressed teens."

Her stepfather worked at a hospital and used to bring home suture kits and needles sometimes. (He would use them for fishing and for his first-aid kit.) She would sneak a needle or a razor blade and use it to carve pentacles and anarchy symbols on her biceps. This was something easily hidden by T-shirts, but also something that she could still show to her best friend and seem "cool."

"I never wanted to kill myself by bleeding to death," she added. "I really just liked the feeling of the pain—the way it made me focus on myself absolutely and completely, on the thoughts and emotions I was having, instead of being distracted by everyday happenings like school, chores, siblings. I liked the knowledge that the body could feel so much pain, since I didn't think I could feel anything at all. I was numb, or at least I wanted to be most of the time so people around me wouldn't be able to take advantage of me. I could now have control over my own feelings and no one else could hurt them."

Shannon soon started writing dirty stories about her sadomasochistic fantasies and tried to realize them with one of her first boyfriends at the age of eighteen. According to her, he was a moody bastard, hated himself for hurting her, and eventually wouldn't do it anymore. "That sucked," is how she summed it up.

A few years later, in the early 2000s, Shannon did something I wouldn't necessarily recommend, but which led her down the path to BDSM: She joined an online chat room. There she met someone she could really just let go with. In her words, she could be "100 percent at his mercy."

After "online spanking sessions," they arranged a meeting, and he told her exactly what to wear. He drove to her college and they met in person in a public space. They were actually attracted to each other and they had lunch (where he made her sit on the chair bare-assed). Every move she made, he orchestrated. She wasn't allowed to even smile without his permission. "By the time lunch came to the table, I was dripping wet," she added.

Long story short, they eventually went to a hotel (also not a great idea if you've just met a person) and had an encounter that changed her life. "I was literally giving myself over to someone else and it felt like heaven," Shannon said. "I don't know how else to describe it, but it really was transcendent. He wanted to utterly own me and I allowed that in order to feel like I knew myself. It was very sexual, of course, but it was also spiritual. It was like giving your life over to a deity and letting him/her know you were ready to do anything they wanted as long as they guide you toward personal freedom. Up until then, I had never felt more beautiful than at that moment. I felt whole for once in my life, with nothing to worry about—no chores or tests or work schedules could possibly break into my thoughts to distract me. I was purely held in those unfolding moments; for that period of time, my entire body was present, my mind was present, and my spirit felt like it was truly where it wanted to be."

I've since learned that this is the way people often describe enlightenment. You might not "see God," but you could very well experience a feeling of "Life is simple! I can do this!" Much like deeply meditating, creating a work of art, or even having a great meal can make you forget about everyday bullshit, so can BDSM.

By the way, "Shannon" asked that I change her name for the book because she still fears judgment. Admitting you're kinky, that you like to be tied up or spanked, or that you like to do the tying up and spanking and everything else in between takes courage. I hope reading this book gives people the courage to let their freak flags fly. This is why I've admitted to so many nutty things herein—because at the end of the day, for every person that doesn't love me because I'm a "freak," there is someone who will love me more (and more honestly) for just being real.

It's funny how sometimes those who espouse the "don't judge lest ye be judged" mantra are so quick to do it anyway. As far as I can see, when practiced ethically, BDSM gives people a chance to explore three things that keep the world in motion: love, sex, and power. These may be part of the true meaning of the "three legs" on O's ring. There would be no "man's progress" without them.

The Difference between BDSM and Abuse

Sadly, as much fun as BDSM can be, the fact is that some people will use it as a cover for abusive behavior. *Consent* must always be part of whatever is happening. Again, as a Dom, be sure that you are not consenting to do anything insane. From a sub's perspective, be wary of any partner who will not stop what's happening at any time even when you say your safe word.

You should not only be able to withdraw consent, but also be able to express limits and needs without being ridiculed, criticized, or coerced into changing them. Your partner should not threaten to "out" you for being into BDSM or for being polyamorous or gay. And a Dom should never attempt to convince you to do anything illegal.

The terms of BDSM play are always negotiated ahead of time. Abuse isn't. There are rules in BDSM. In abuse, there are no rules. An abuser will try to keep you from being near friends and family, whereas BDSM can happen in social scenes and at parties (*some* social scenes and *some* parties).

If you find yourself isolated and caught up in an abusive relationship, there are places where you can get help, regain your power, and get on with your life. The National Domestic Violence Hotline (800) 799-7233 is a good place to start, but there are plenty of other resources and support groups online.

BDSM is all about love, even if it stings, burns, or sometimes bruises! And this brings us to the final portion of the book, where stinging is most likely to occur—the end.

The End

Where else could I end but at *the* end? The rear end, the bottom, the buttocks, or derriere—whatever name you give it, the ass is a vital part of BDSM and this is the ass-end of this book. If you ask me, all asses—big and small, flat and buoyant, square and heart-shaped—bring pleasure to the world. They are spanked, licked, massaged, worshipped, erotically tortured, and plugged with butt plugs and penises. Overall, they are just fun.

I am sorry that in this book we never covered cock and ball torture or advanced hog-tying methods. We hardly even discussed my favorite thing: outfits.

One word of advice when it comes to outfits, specifically corsets:

Avoid shelf-boob, as it is the bane of Ren Faires everywhere. Get one that fits properly and won't cinch you so hard you pass out. Orchard Corsetry, a store in my neighborhood on the Lower East Side, is the best undergarment store in the world. If you ever get a chance, visit and meet the "bra whisperer."

Also, in terms of outfits, don't spend a lot of money. One simple black thong can do wonders. Of course, being retired, I only wear granny panties these days.

Corsets, thongs, and cock and ball torture aside, this is a starter guide and luckily there are a million books out there specializing in these subjects. Let's get back to ass.

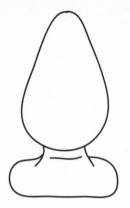

At this point, you should know what to do with the ass. Don't misuse a cornucopia of vegetables in it—really nothing from the produce aisle—unless you want to go trick-or-treating at the ER. And, if what's going in there is something other than a penis, make sure it has a flared base. There are so many fine butt plugs out there, some of which vibrate, so have fun with toys. (Mr. Hall even told me a story about tying a thin rope to a butt plug, which he then inserted into his partner and used to guide her while she gave him oral. He certainly gets an A+ for creativity here.)

As with everything else in BDSM, when dealing with the ass, go slowly. Tell your partners that you adore them, that you want their asses and that you would do anything to touch them, spank them, whatever your pleasure. In other words, kiss their asses.

And, adore your own ass, as it will be tagging along behind you throughout your whole life. Learn to enjoy your ass, the "middle child of the penis and vagina." (It acts up!) Be kind to it and to your body. If you need a massage, ask for one. If you want a spanking, ask for one. And if you need a kiss or a hug, I suppose it's okay to ask for one of those things, too.

In all seriousness, though I am juvenile enough to end a book with "the end," I can recognize one simple truth about BDSM:

While it is about pleasure, pain, and kink, one humanistic principle should reign supreme throughout—kindness. Be very nice to whomever you are about to fuck, spank, whip, or flog. Earn your sub's devotion and trust. And as a sub, know that you have control, that nothing is ever out of your hands even when your hands are tied behind your back. If you're picky in your partners and strict about safety, you may find more than just a play partner. You may find a friend and lover for life.

Acknowledgments

There are many people to thank for the making of this book.

First, I offer gratitude to anyone who's ever covered this subject with an open mind and to readers for being brave sexual explorers. I wish you all a happy, transcendent journey full of chips, dips, chains, and whips.

Second, to my friends Scooter Pie, Faceboy, Amanda, Stormy, Velocity, and many more: Thank you for sharing your expertise, knowledge, and openness.

To my agent, Jennifer Lyons, thank you for working on my behalf and thanks to Skyhorse for putting this book out there.

To my partner, Courtney, I offer thanks for accepting my writing benders and my perverse sense of fun.

Rock on, people.

Notes

Chains, Whips, and Cuffs

_____

_____

_____

_____

_____

_____

_____

_____

_____

_____

_____

_____

_____

_____

ALSO AVAILABLE

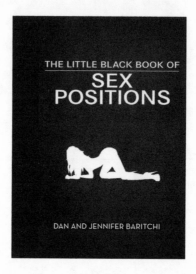

The Little Black Book of Sex Positions
by Dan and Jennifer Baritchi

If you think there are only three positions that get the job done, then it's time to get out of your sexual rut and start having a ball! *The Little Black Book of Sex Positions* exposes in glorious detail hundreds of sexy moves that can lead to mind-blowing ecstasy for you and your lover. The positions offered here are the next best thing to having an experienced partner right by your side . . . or behind, or face-to-face.

If your rolls in the hay have become a bit ho-hum, or if you just want to expand your spicy repertoire, this hot little how-to will having you flexing muscles you never knew you had with sexy positions you've always wanted to try like the YMCA, Forbidden Fruit, Pirate's Bounty, Rodeo, Deep Impact, and much more.

In a hardcover edition with full-color exciting yet tasteful illustrations, *The Little Black Book of Sex Positions* is handsome enough to keep on your nightstand, or to give to someone naughty and nice. You'll never think about "little black book" the same way again. Start stretching!

$16.95 Hardcover • ISBN 978-1-62087-611-4

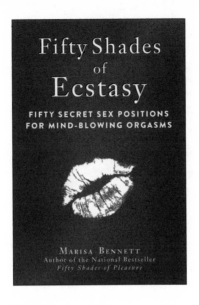

Fifty Shades of Ecstasy
Fifty Secret Sex Positions for Mind-Blowing Orgasms
by Marisa Bennett

If the latest wave of popular erotic romance has gotten your motor running, this book will shift you into high gear!

Author Marisa Bennett steps up again to give you the dirty details on doing the horizontal hula, with wit, humor, and some hot new moves. This guide will help you expand your sexual repertoire and hone your sexytime skills while exploring ecstasy in fifty (count 'em, fifty!) different ways. You'll learn a ton of fun and sexy positions like the visually-stimulating Pin-Up Girl, the cozy Lock and Key, and the hot and creative Bobsled (also known as "sledding on Bob"), each one beautifully illustrated to help make sure you've got everything in the proper place.

So what are you waiting for? Whether you are single and ready to (co)mingle or married and want to put some new moves into your old routine, pick up this hot how-to and kick your sexcapades up to the next level with fifty new ways to get it on.

$12.95 Hardcover • ISBN 978-1-61608-755-5

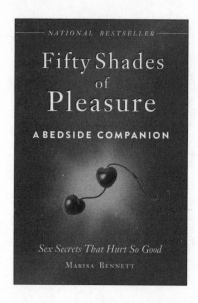

Fifty Shades of Pleasure: A Bedside Companion
Sex Secrets That Hurt So Good

by Marisa Bennett

If hot erotic romance novels have had you fantasizing about certain naughty pleasures, or if you just want to add a little spice to your sexy love sessions, this kinky how-to will bring your fantasies to life. Explore the pleasure of a little pain, flex muscles you didn't know you had through hot sex positions, and learn how to make or break the rules in your playtime romp.

With a light, playful tone, this book eases you into the stingingly sweet side of sex. Each section features excerpts from the Kama Sutra or classic erotica, extra tips like "Dirty Talk Dos and Dont's," and further resources to continue your naughty education. Gather your ben wa balls and feather ticklers while this handbook gives you the rundown on all the hot moves you've been wanting to try, from beginner bondage techniques and starter spanking to hot wax and flogging—no dungeon required!

$12.95 Hardcover • ISBN 978-1-62087-334-2

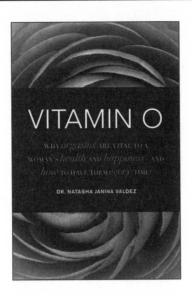

Vitamin O
Why Orgasms are Vital to a Woman's Health and Happiness—and How to Have Them Every Time!
by Dr. Natasha Janina Valdez

They're free, fun, and with this book, easy to achieve.

Far too many women aren't enjoying the benefits of this delicious activity, and Dr. Natasha wants to change that. In *Vitamin O*, she explores manual techniques, oral methods, and crazy-fun sex positions that maximize a woman's pleasure. She covers the basics in orgasmic foreplay, orgasmic positions, exercises to improve orgasms, orgasm-enhancing yoga, breathing techniques, and more. Here is the 411 on more advanced climaxing—multiples and simultaneous orgasms. And she breaks out lots of quick fixes for getting a daily dose without any fuss. By the time she's through, having orgasms will become as natural and pleasantly habitual as drinking a morning coffee (which you'll be drinking less and less of, as you'll have increased energy from better sleep).

Vitamin O's benefits are layered and far-reaching, without any worry of toxicity or build-up—because Vitamin O is all about release. Regular doses will benefit every reader for life.

$14.95 Paperback • ISBN 978-1-61608-311-3